SCHIZOPHRENIA IN THE 21ST CENTURY

Edited by **T.H.J. Burne**

Schizophrenia in the 21st Century
Edited by T.H.J. Burne

Published by InTech

Janeza Trdine 9, 51000 Rijeka, Croatia

Publishing Process Manager Petra Nenadic

Technical Editor Teodora Smiljanic

Cover Designer InTech Design Team

Additional hard copies can be obtained from orders@intechopen.com

Schizophrenia in the 21st Century, Edited by T.H.J. Burne
p. cm.
ISBN 978-953-51-0315-8

For EU product safety concerns:
IN TECH d.o.o., Prolaz Marije Krucifikse Kozulić 3, 51000 Rijeka, Croatia,
info@intechopen.com or visit our website at intechopen.com.

Meet the editor

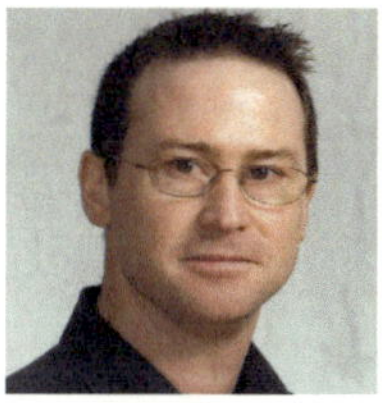

Dr Burne obtained his PhD in Behavioural Neuroscience and he is active in research on brain development and behaviour in animal models to learn more about neuropsychiatric diseases. His research is focused on investigating the underlying biological basis for schizophrenia, with the goal of finding public health interventions that will alleviate the burden of this disease. Dr Burne is part of the Queensland Centre for Mental Health Research and has been situated within the Queensland Brain Institute since 2005. He has published over 70 refereed papers and book chapters, is an Academic Editor for PLoS One and on the executive committee for the Australasian Society for Psychiatric Research.

Contents

Preface

This book began as a collection of articles on neuropsychiatric disease, but with a clear focus on Schizophrenia, which is a poorly understood but very disabling group of brain disorders. We now recognize schizophrenia as a disorder of the brain, but despite advances in treatment options we are still a long way from having effective treatments, particularly for cognitive symptoms, and lack effective interventions and ways to prevent this disease. While hallucinations and delusions (*positive symptoms* of schizophrenia) feature prominently in diagnostic criteria, impairments of memory and attentional processing (*cognitive symptoms* of schizophrenia) are attracting increasing interest in modern neuropsychiatry. *Schizophrenia in the 21st Century* gives an overview of current research on schizophrenia (Part I) and brings together various aspects of clinical research into cognitive symptoms (Part II) and preclinical research in animal models (Part III).

Prof. Robert Hunter provides an up to date review of "Treatment of schizophrenia in the 21st Century". There is a major focus on treatments with antipsychotic medications and despite advances in neuroscience of schizophrenia, there is still a need for more effective and safer drugs. However, there is still a place for community-based systems of care, inpatient services, rehabilitation and psycho-social interventions. In the next chapter Dr Setsuko Hanzawa offers an insight into attitudes towards the unique aspects of family caregivers of people with schizophrenia in Japan and Korea, in "Family caregivers of people with schizophrenia in East Asian countries".

There are a number of chapters covering various aspects of cognitive symptoms of schizophrenia in Part II. Luciana de Carvalho Monteiro and colleagues present an overview of schizophrenia and social cognition and suggest that deficits in social cognition are observed throughout the course of schizophrenia. Despite pharmacological and cognitive rehabilitation treatments more research is required to clarify their impact on social cognition. Following along this theme Drs Rafael Penadés and Rosa Catalán examine cognitive remediation therapy to improve neurocognitive outcomes in schizophrenia. Given that cognitive deficits are more closely linked to functional outcomes than psychiatric symptoms there is a clear need for novel psychological interventions. Dr Martin Vargas and colleagues continue this theme providing an overview on metacognitive dysfunction in schizophrenia, which broadly covers deficits in metarepresentation and executive function. The next chapter by Drs

McAllindon and Tibbo examines response selection slowing as a fundamental aspect of the cognitive deficits of schizophrenia, presenting a detailed review of neuroimaging studies of response selection in healthy controls and in people with schizophrenia. Response selection slowing has a long history in schizophrenia research and may be an endophenotype of schizophrenia, although the promise of new medications for effective treatments seems a long way off.

Preclincal research into schizophrenia is the focus of Part III. Drs Tomiki Sumiyoshi and Takashi Uehara specifically address a novel hypothesis linking brain energy metabolism and disturbances of cognition function, providing evidence for serotinergic receptors as promising candidates for cognitive enhancers. In the next chapter Professor Jones reviews the literature on animal models used to study schizophrenia, with a particular focus on animal models with disruptions to the hippocampus and the thalamus. The final chapter by Stuchlik and colleagues covers a range of behavioural tests in rodent animal models that are used to evaluate information processing and cognitive deficits of relevance to neuropsychiatric disorders. Although it is not possible to recapitulate all of the features of schizophrenia in an animal model, preclinical research using animal models is a powerful tool in understanding the neuroscience of higher cognitive functions and the discovery of novel drugs aimed at restoring normal cognitive function.

Schizophrenia is a debilitating group of disorders and there is much work to be done before we understand the neuroscience of schizophrenia and have safe and effective treatments for all patients. Antipsychotic drugs have largely been effective at treating the positive symptoms of schizophrenia. However, we do not have adequate treatments for cognitive dysfunction, which is a core part of the disorder. This book provides the reader with a diversity of findings examining a range of available treatment options into cognitive symptoms with evidence presented from both clinical and preclinical studies.

Dr. T.H.J. Burne
Queensland Brain Institute,
The University of Queensland,
Australia

Part 1

Schizophrenia in the 21st Century

1

Treatment of Schizophrenia in the 21st Century: Towards a more Personalised Approach

Robert Hunter
University of Glasgow
Institute of Neuroscience and Psychology
Gartnavel Royal Hospital, Glasgow
UK

1. Introduction

'Canst thou not minister to a mind diseased, pluck from the memory a rooted sorrow, raze out the written troubles of the brain, and with some sweet oblivious antidote cleanse the fraught bosom of that perilous stuff which weighs upon the heart?'
Macbeth, William Shakespeare

'You look at where you're going and where you are and it never makes sense, but then you look back at where you've been and a pattern seems to emerge. And if you project forward from that pattern, then sometimes you can come up with something'
Zen and the Art of Motorcycle Maintenance, Robert Pirsig

What are the prospects for advances in the treatment of schizophrenia as the 21st Century unfolds? It is clear that many advances have been made in the 100 years since Eugen Bleuler's important monograph *Dementia Praecox or the Group of Schizophrenias*, compiled detailed clinical descriptions of his asylum patients (Bleuler 1911; 1950). Bleuler is remembered for introducing the term schizophrenia, in preference to Kraepelin's dementia praecox, but his monograph is an exemplar of comprehensive psychopathological description, and as the title of the monograph suggests, Bleuler conceived that schizophrenia was a group of conditions, rather a single nosological entity.

Although advances have undoubtedly occurred, considered reflections about the seminal contributions of Bleuler - and indeed Kraepelin - in this centenary year, may make one wonder whether these treatment advances are a somewhat thin veneer, rather than the step change required. It could be argued that progress has been more due to changes in societal values and attitudes rather than the development of effective novel interventions – either pharmacological or psychological.

We are unfortunately still some way off from understanding the neuroscience of this family of disorders, and developing rational therapies built on that understanding. It is indisputable that the antipsychotic medication of today is essentially a variant of pharmacology developed through serendipitous discovery 50 years ago. Thus in the second decade of the 21st Century, the 'Dopamine Hypothesis' is still the dominant paradigm, and a newly introduced antipsychotic (asenapine) - with dopaminergic pharmacology - is the new kid in town. Yet exciting advances in neuroscience have, and are being made, and slowly but surely we are taking small steps forward to understand the brain. But for those of us impatient to have better treatments and interventions sooner rather than later, these scientific advances, seem too small and too slow. Take molecular genetics and bioinformatics for example; these are perhaps two of the most exciting areas of biology and are beginning to have an impact on other areas of medical therapeutics such as cancer and diabetes, and provide a signpost to 'personalised medicine'. Yet recent genome wide association (GWAS) studies of large samples, have demonstrated that in schizophrenia around 1000 or more genetic variants of low penetrance may be implicated in the heritability of schizophrenia. The crux of the schizophrenia enigma is that we are dealing with a complex family of disorders affecting the most complex of cognitive functions, namely information processing. Whatever else it is, the genus schizophrenia is hugely complex but future treatments should benefit from an explosion of findings in basic and clinical neuroscience, provided they can be translated into new therapies.

The World Health Organisation (WHO) estimates that schizophrenia, depression, epilepsy, dementia, alcohol dependence and other mental, neurological and substance-use (MNS) disorders constitute 13% of the global burden of disease, surpassing both cardiovascular disease and cancer (WHO 2008). Worldwide, schizophrenia is 3rd highest ranked MNS disorder after depression (1st) and Alcohol-use disorders (2nd), considerably higher than epilepsy (7th) and Parkinson's disease (13th) (see Table 1). The amount of health lost because

Table 1. The global burden of mental, neurological and substance use (MNS) disorders*

	Worldwide		High income countries**		Low- and middle-income countries	
Rank	Cause	DALYs*** (millions)	Cause	DALYs (millions)	Cause	DALYs (millions)
1	Unipolar depressive disorders	65.5	Unipolar depressive disorders	10.0	Unipolar depressive disorders	55.5
2	Alcohol use disorders	23.7	Alzheimer's & other dementias	4.4	Alcohol use disorders	19.5
3	Schizophrenia	16.8	Alcohol use disorders	4.2	Schizophrenia	15.2
4	Bipolar affective disorder	14.4	Drug-use disorders	1.9	Bipolar affective disorder	12.9
5	Alzheimer's & other dementias	11.2	Schizophrenia	1.6	Epilepsy	7.3
6	Drug-use disorders	8.4	Bipolar affective disorder	1.5	Alzheimer's & other dementias	6.8
7	Epilepsy	7.9	Migraine	1.4	Drug-use disorders	6.5
8	Migraine	7.8	Panic disorder	0.8	Migraine	6.3
9	Panic disorder	7.0	Insomnia (primary)	0.8	Panic disorder	6.2
10	Obsessive compulsive disorder	5.1	Parkinson's disease	0.7	Obsessive compulsive disorder	4.5
11	Insomnia (primary)	3.6	Obsessive compulsive disorder	0.6	Post-traumatic stress disorder	3.0
12	Post-traumatic stress disorder	3.5	Epilepsy	0.5	Insomnia (primary)	2.9
13	Parkinson's disease	1.7	Post-traumatic stress disorder	0.5	Multiple sclerosis	1.2
14	Multiple sclerosis	1.5	Multiple sclerosis	0.3	Parkinson's disease	1.0

*Examples of MNS disorders under the purview of the Grand Challenges in Global Mental Health Initiative.
**World Bank criteria for income (2009 gross national income (GNI) per capita): low income is US $995 equivalent or less; middle income is $996-12995; high income is $12996 or more.
***A disability-adjusted life year (DALY) is a unit for measuring the amount of health lost because of a disease or injury. It is calculated as the present value of the future years of disability-free life that are lost as a result of the premature deaths or disability occurring in a particular year.

Reprinted with thanks from Collins et al (2011) Grand challenges in global mental health. Nature 475, 27-30.

MIS 249643

Table 1. The global burden of mental, neurological and substance-use (MNS) disorders.

of a disease or injury can be best estimated using Disability-Adjusted Life Years (DALY) which is calculated as the present value of the future years of disability-free life that are lost as a result of the premature deaths or disability occurring in a particular year. As shown in Table 1, schizophrenia accounts for 16.8 million DALYs on a global basis, ranging from ~1.6m to ~16m for high and low income countries respectively. The economic and social consequences of mental ill health are considerable and impact differently on developed and developing countries. The drain on national wealth is highly significant;

for example the social and economic costs of mental illness in Scotland were recently calculated at 8% of GDP perhaps around £10b sterling (SAMH, 2007).

In this chapter I will review the current status of treatment for schizophrenia in terms of effectiveness and safety, and discuss what treatment advances have been made in the last century, and how treatment interventions might and should develop as the 21st century unfolds. The emphasis of the chapter will be on pharmacological treatment and the scope for new drugs, but I will also discuss briefly the place of community systems of care, the role of inpatient services, rehabilitation and recovery models, and to a much lesser degree I will also discuss the developing role of psycho-social interventions.

2. Clinical considerations

The lifetime prevalence of schizophrenia is approximately 1% (0.70 - 1.10%) and incidence rates vary from 0.2 to 0.7 (Picchioni & Murray 2007; McGrath 2006). The onset of symptoms typically occurs in early adult life (average age 25 years), and occurs earlier in men than in women (Aleman, 2003). Schizophrenia is characterised by three key symptom domains: *positive symptoms*, such as auditory hallucinations, delusions, and thought disorder; *negative symptoms*, including anhedonia, social withdrawal, affective flattening, and demotivation; and *cognitive dysfunction*, particularly in the domains of attention, working memory, and executive function (Tamminga & Holcomb 2005). Schizophrenia is typically a life-long condition characterised by acute symptom exacerbations and widely varying degrees of functional disability. About 25% of people with schizophrenia are resistant to treatment with antipsychotic medication; treatment resistance is usually defined as a lack of clinically important improvement in symptoms, usually positive symptoms, after 2 to 3 regimens of treatment with standard antipsychotic drugs for at least 6 weeks. Of those people with schizophrenia who do benefit from antipsychotic medication, an additional 30% to 40% are residually symptomatic despite adequate antipsychotic treatment (Kane et al 1988).

About three-quarters of people with schizophrenia suffer recurrent relapses and continued disability. Outcome appears to be worse in people with the following factors: 1) an insidious onset of symptoms where initial treatment is delayed; 2) social isolation; 3) a strong family history of schizophrenia or other major mental disorder; 4) people living in industrialised countries and urbanised communities; 5) men appear to fair worse than women; and 6) in those people who misuse drugs especially cannabis, and possibly from an early age under 16 years (Jablensky et al 1992). Drug treatment is generally more successful in treating positive symptoms, but up to one third of people derive little benefit, and negative symptoms are notoriously difficult to treat. Adherence to treatment plans appears to be a particular challenge in schizophrenia due to many factors but including reduced or absent insight into the nature of their mental change. About half of people with schizophrenia do not adhere to treatment in the short term and adherence is even lower in the longer term (Johnstone, 1993).

The term schizophrenia is of course rather imprecise, and is defined clinically rather than on the basis of any biopathological markers and refers to a spectrum or family of psychotic disorders, with a range of clinical phenotypes. This clinical heterogeneity will be familiar to all clinicians treating people with 'schizophrenia', but within the spectrum of schizophrenic illness the classification systems of ICD10 (WHO) and DSM4 (APA) help provide reasonable reliability about diagnosis, at least in general terms. Risk factors associated with the aetiology of schizophrenia include the following: 1) a positive family history (reflecting at least in part genetic factors); 2) obstetric complications; 3) developmental difficulties; 4) central nervous system infections or other insults in childhood; 5) cannabis use; and 6) acutely traumatic life events (McGrath, 2006). The precise contributions of these factors, and ways in which they may interact, are unclear. For example, the heritability of schizophrenia has been estimated to be as high as 81% and recent genome wide association (GWAS) studies of large sample size, demonstrate that the clinical heterogeneity of schizophrenia probably reflects, a complex biological heterogeneity (Sullivan et al 2003). GWAS studies suggest that probably ~1000 genetic variants of low penetrance (Purcell et al 2009; Shi et al 2009; Stefansson et al 2009) and other individually rare genetic variants of higher penetrance, along with epigenetic mechanisms are responsible, *pari passu* with environmental factors, such as those above, in contributing to a complex and varied clinical phenotype. The lack of understanding of the mechanisms whereby the above aetiological factors (genetic and environmental) interact to initiate the complex pathobiology of schizophrenia is the key reason for the relative lack of progress in the development of novel drug treatments. All the antipsychotic medication that is currently in use (first and second generation) is all predicated on the so-called 'Dopamine Hypothesis' (discussed below) and share a common putative mechanism of action, namely dopamine antagonism. The benefits of 'major tranquilisers' such as chlorpromazine were first observed in the 1950s by serendipity rather than from a rational understanding of the key drug targets needed to treat schizophrenia. Unfortunately fifty years later we still await a new class of antipsychotics that have a mechanism of action predicated on advances in understanding the neuroscience of the condition.

3. Pharmacotherapy

Increasing evidence suggests that serious mental illness is neurodevelopmental and the onset of pre-psychotic symptoms occurs in adolescence, at a time when the cerebral cortex is still developing. As with many complex disorders (e.g. hypertension, epilepsy, and diabetes), there appear to be many aetiological pathways that might lead to the final mixture of behavioral signs and symptoms we label 'schizophrenia'. If there is general agreement that the key symptom domains present in schizophrenia: positive, negative, cognitive and affective, are a priority for treatment, then to what extent do currently available antipsychotic drugs succeed in ameliorating such symptoms and difficulties? Another important question is how well tolerated are the available drugs and what adverse effects are associated with them? In addressing these questions it is important to understand that the evidence base of randomised controlled trials (RCTs) that we might use to address these issues has been generated almost entirely by the pharmaceutical industry for the purpose of obtaining a license to market a particular therapeutic moiety in a particular jurisdiction. Another pitfall that is worth being aware of, is a tendency to accept the results of systematic reviews uncritically. While many such reviews can be useful, they reflect the sum of their parts; if the constituent studies are defective then misleading summary statistics may result. Furthermore such RCTs almost always, with one or two notable exceptions, provide information about efficacy rather than effectiveness in 'real world' rather than idealised, clinical settings and rarely provide information about cost benefit analysis. There are of course exceptions to this, but in general these are the exception rather than the rule. So with this important caveat in mind, what can we conclude about the efficacy of the current licensed medicinal products?

We have recently completed a thorough review of the published literature of RCT evidence for BMJ Clinical Evidence (Barry et al 2012). In preparing this review for *Clinical Evidence* of the clinical trial literature for interventions for schizophrenia, a comprehensive search strategy identified all relevant publications, and those studies meeting reasonable quality standards were then included as described. Despite such a careful triage process, that aimed to include only good quality RCTs, it is clear that many studies we included have serious failings. Moreover, and perhaps surprisingly, objective assessment of the available evidence base for the efficacy of antipsychotic medication (and other interventions) is much less convincing than one would have hoped. Common issues being: small underpowered studies, sample bias, less than transparent methodology and data analysis, inappropriate outcome measures, to name but a few. Although in many trials haloperidol has been used as the standard comparator, the clinical trial evidence for haloperidol itself is much less impressive than one might expect (Barry et al 2012). By their very nature systematic reviews and RCTs provide only *average* indices of probable *efficacy* in groups of individuals recruited to the study in question. Although many RCTs attempt to limit inclusion criteria to a single category of diagnosis from DSM4 or ICD10, many studies include individuals with different types of schizophrenic diagnosis such as schizoaffective disorder. In all RCTs, even those recruiting according to DSM-4 or ICD10 diagnoses, there will still be considerable clinical heterogeneity, as will be recognised by clinicians treating people with 'schizophrenia' or psychotic conditions.

Clearly a more *stratified* approach to clinical trials would help identify those subgroups who appear to be the best responders to a particular intervention. To date however there is little to suggest that stratification on the basis of clinical characteristics successfully helps predict which drugs work best for which patients. There is a pressing need for the development of biomarkers with clinical utility, for mental health problems. Such measures could help stratify clinical populations or provide better markers of efficacy in clinical trials, and would complement the current use of clinical outcome scales. Clinicians are also well aware that many patients treated with antipsychotic medication, develop significant and particular adverse effects such as EPS or weight gain. Again our ability to identify which patients will develop which adverse effects is poorly developed, and might be assisted by employing biomarkers to stratify patient populations. In future the use of biomarkers that can be used in the clinic to help determine diagnostic response groups will represent an important advance.

Another important consideration is that the DSM-4 which has so dominated interventional research in schizophrenia for many years may have inadvertently inhibited drug development. Although the DSM-4 includes negative symptoms, the diagnostic criteria for schizophrenia can still be met in patients with hallucinations and/or delusions alone, without the other symptoms associated with the disorder. As a result people included in trials have constituted a rather heterogeneous clinical group. This may have resulted a bias towards the development of treatments for positive (reality distortion) symptoms and compromised the discovery of interventions for negative or cognitive symptoms: potentially another reason for the paucity of effective therapeutics. These considerations are reflected in the support for DSM-5 to include dimensions of pychopathology in addition to diagnostic class (http://www.dsm5.org). If implemented in DSM-5, there may well be a requirement for symptom domains such as depression, anxiety, thought disorder, negative and cognition to be assessed. As discussed above this could improve drug development and afford better opportunities for psychopathology to be mapped onto neural substrates as proposed in the NIMH Research Diagnostic Criteria initiative (Cuthbert & Insel 2010). These authors have discussed in detail how 'the inertia of diagnostic orthodoxy has exerted a powerful hegemony over any alternative approaches, leaving us with much debate but little data with which to construct a new nosology'.

3.1 First and second-generation antipsychotics

The results of the BMJ Clinical Evidence review tend to indicate that as far as antipsychotic medication goes, current drugs are of some, if limited, efficacy in many patients, and that most drugs cause side effects in most patients. Although this is a rather downbeat conclusion, this will not be too surprising to clinicians in the field, given their clinical experience and our knowledge of the pharmacology of the available antipsychotic medication. Currently available antipsychotic medication has the same putative mechanism of action namely, dopaminergic antagonism with varying degrees of antagonism at other receptor sites that appear to modulate the appearance of a range of adverse consequences. More efficacious antipsychotic medication awaits a better understanding of the biological pathogenesis of these conditions so that rational therapies can be developed.

First line, standard treatment of schizophrenia and related psychotic illness is with antipsychotic drugs. All members of this drug class appear to exert their antipsychotic effect through dopaminergic antagonism. The first such drugs to be introduced included chlorpromazine and haloperidol, members of the drug group now referred to as 'first generation antipsychotics' (FGA). Chlorpromazine was synthesized in December 1951 in the laboratories of Rhône-Poulenc, and became available on prescription in France in November 1952. Its effectiveness was reflected in the transformation of disturbed wards; its commercial success stimulated the development of other psychotropic drugs (Delay, Deniker & Harl, 1952). As is well known FGA can cause severe adverse effects such as extra-pyramidal side effects including Parkinsonism and acute dystonia, as well as hyperprolactinaemia and sedation. Attempts to address these adverse effects led to the development of second-generation antipsychotics (SGA). When the SGA were introduced they were commonly known as 'atypical antipsychotics' to distinguish them from the FGA; the terms FGA and SGA are to be preferred as they infer less about the nature of the compound. The systematic review for BMJ Clinical Evidence (Barry et al 2012) summarises a considerable body of evidence from many RCTs and systematic reviews. This shows that the second-generation antipsychotics, amisulpride, clozapine, olanzapine and risperidone appear to be more effective than FGA drugs at reducing positive symptoms, and may cause similar adverse effects, but are associated with additional concerns about metabolic effects such as weight gain, impaired glucose tolerance and hyperlipidaemia. Antipsychotics such as pimozide, quetiapine, aripiprazole, sulpiride, ziprasidone and zotepine appear to be as effective as standard antipsychotic drugs in improving positive symptoms. But again, these drugs can cause adverse effects in some patients similar to other FGA and SGA drugs. It should be noted that the use of pimozide has been associated with sudden cardiac death at doses above 20 mg daily. Antipsychotic maintenance treatment reduces relapse rates from 54% to 20% within approximately 10 months (absolute risk difference (ARD) = 37%; relative risk reduction (RRR) = 66% weighted) which translates as a NNT of 3, which is considered a large effect size (Leucht et al 2011).

It is worth emphasising however that we now appear to have a range of compounds that in some patients at least, and for some time, help to control positive psychotic symptoms. While this is very important, this benefit may come with associated adverse consequences in other ways for some patients, such as cardio-metabolic side effects that can have a major impact on physical health. Clinicians therefore will need to exercise careful and skilled judgement about which antipsychotic to use in order to benefit individual patient's symptoms, and minimise adverse health effects. There is real scope for the pharmaceutical industry to develop new drugs for positive symptoms - perhaps dopaminergic antagonists - that are less toxic and prone to cause adverse health effects.

As noted above data from trials provides little help in gauging how an individual patient will respond to or suffer from any one treatment. It has become apparent in recent years that a priority area for psychiatrists must be to ensure that the physical health of patients is monitored and addressed, given that patients with schizophrenia often have significant chronic co-morbidities such as diabetes and heart disease.

There is limited evidence to indicate whether any antipsychotic other than clozapine is effective in people with treatment-resistant schizophrenia. In people resistant to standard antipsychotic drugs, clozapine may improve symptoms compared with other first-generation and second generation antipsychotic agents, but this benefit must be balanced against the likelihood of important adverse effects such as neutropaenia, cardio-metabolic effects and sedation. It is also worth stating that quoted estimates of the prevalence of treatment resistance (around 25%) are likely to be a considerable underestimate. In the Scottish Schizophrenia Outcomes Study (Hunter et al 2009), 40% of a representative sample of 1000 people attending services with ICD10 schizophrenia, were prescribed clozapine, which could be considered a proxy for treatment resistance.

3.2 Negative symptoms and cognitive impairment

While there is evidence of efficacy of antipsychotics with respect to positive symptoms, there is much less evidence of benefit of these agents on negative symptoms. Negative symptoms were first described by Kraepelin in 1919 as the 'avolitional syndrome' (Kraepelin 1919) and the term now refers to the absence or reduction in normal behaviours and functions (Mäkinen et al 2008) Negative symptoms are listed from the PANSS Negative Subscale in Table 2. Persistent negative symptoms can be either primary or secondary and usually persist during periods of clinical stability, when positive symptoms may have remitted and they often interfere with the ability to perform normal everyday functions.

Negative and cognitive symptoms are important areas where the drugs currently available have only minimal benefit and patients have considerable unmet need (Kirkpatrick 2006; NICE 2011).

N1 Blunted affect
N2 Emotional withdrawal
N3 Poor rapport
N4 Passive / apathetic social withdrawal
N5 Difficulty in abstract thinking
N6 lack of spontaneity and flow of conversation
N7 Stereotyped thinking

Table 2. Positive and Negative Symptom Scale - Negative Subscale.

A substantial number of studies now show that the severity of cognitive impairments in people with schizophrenia is predictive of getting back to meaningful activity, perhaps work, social functioning and independent living (Green 1996). Increased recognition of this is the key reason for the burgeoning interest in Neurocognition as a target for either pharmacological or psychological intervention strategies ('cognitive remediation' for example see Wykes & Spaulding 2011).

In the BMJ Clinical Evidence review (Barry et al 2012), we were unable to reach conclusions about the effect of antipsychotic drugs on cognitive symptoms due to a lack of RCTs and the lack of standardized validated measures in available trials. This is clearly an area that pharma and the research community must address. There are signs again that this is changing. The FDA has recognised the importance of cognitive impairment in schizophrenia and funded development of a clinical cognitive test battery, the MATRICS: Measurement & Treatment Research to Improve Cognition in Schizophrenia (see Buchanan et al 2005 and www.matrics.ucla.edu). The MATRICS comprises seven cognitive domains: Speed of processing, Attention/Vigilance, Working Memory, Verbal Learning & memory, Visual Learning & memory, Problem solving, and Social Cognition. The FDA has recommended that the MATRICS Consensus Cognitive Battery should be used as the standard set of cognitive tests for all clinical trials of potential cognitive enhancers in schizophrenia. This is an important initiative which, although MATRICS may well be over engineered with consequent reduced utility for many patients, has undoubtedly influenced the use of cognition as an outcome measure in clinical trials, and perhaps helped encourage the development of pharmacological cognitive enhancers. The FDA has endorsed both cognitive impairment (Buchanan et al 2005) and negative symptoms (Kirkpatrick et al 2006) as distinct therapeutic targets or domains and this approach has attracted support (e.g. Harvey et al 2006). There is however an alternative view that there is overlap between the constructs, 'negative symptoms' and 'cognitive impairment' in schizophrenia (Laughren & Levin, 2011).

It is recognised that both these domains may be largely, though not exclusively, residual phase phenomena. This has been a relatively neglected phase of the condition when patients' positive symptoms are to some extent attenuated or at least manageable, and the individual would aspire to improve the quality of their lives, but is hampered in this, by residual negative symptoms and cognitive impairments. For these reasons the FDA have now recommended that in all future clinical trials targeting either primary negative symptoms or targeting cognitive impairments, researchers should collect data on both these domains (Laughren & Levin, 2011).

We have shown that negative symptoms as assessed by PANSS are strongly related to psychosocial functioning as assessed by a number of different scales across eleven different European centres (Hunter et al 2011). Given the nature of such negative symptoms and their frequent occurrence in schizophrenia, it is reasonable to assume that negative symptoms are an important causal contribution to reduced psychosocial functioning in schizophrenia. This has important implications for the care of people with schizophrenia. Firstly, given that successful community care will require good or at least, adequate psychosocial functioning, improving negative symptomatology is an essential prerequisite. Secondly, physicians, psychologists, researchers and the pharmaceutical industry need to refocus on this area in order to develop effective treatments. There is some evidence that this is starting to occur (see www.ClinicalTrials.gov) although hampered by a still largely incomplete understanding of the pathogenesis and neurobiology of schizophrenia. There are several novel drugs in development - some Phase 3 Trials - that appear to work by modulating glutamatergic function, that may help negative and neurocognitive symptoms.

4. New drugs for schizophrenia?

The 'dopamine hypothesis of schizophrenia' proposes that excessive subcortical dopamine release, linked to prefrontal cortical dopaminergic dysfunction is central to the pathogenesis of schizophrenia (Van Rossum, 1966). Although all antipsychotics modulate dopamine activity in the brain, via dopaminergic antagonism, there is no incontrovertible evidence that schizophrenia is the result of a primary dopamine abnormality. Dopamine dysregulation is likely to be a 'downstream' or a secondary consequence of the primary biological causes of the condition (Coyle, 2006). Despite these qualifications, the dopamine antagonists have provided considerable benefit to many patients in reducing positive symptoms and there are no licensed antipsychotics as yet which do not have dopaminergic antagonism as a key part of their pharmacological profile. It is clear however that the biological basis of schizophrenia is likely to be complex and much more than a dysregulation of dopamine metabolism. As already mentioned GWAS studies sign post several different areas of cellular metabolism that appear involved in pathogenesis and help identify new candidate genes as putative drug targets. For example, the gene *KCNH2* was identified in a large meta-analysis of five independent data sets to be associated with schizophrenia. The *KCNH2* gene encodes a membrane-spanning potassium channel and the expression of *KCNH2-3.1* is specifically increased within the hippocampal formation of individuals with schizophrenia and in normal individuals who carry risk-associated alleles (Huffaker et al, 2009). Genetic linkage and association studies have also implicated members of the Neuregulin-ErbB receptor (NRG-ErbB) signalling pathway as risk factors for schizophrenia (Buonanno et al, 2010). These examples are cited simply to illustrate how genetic studies can help identify genes or groups of genes associated with schizophrenia, and how by understanding the functional significance of such genes we may discover new drug targets.

There is increasing interest in a 'glutamate hypothesis' of schizophrenia that postulates a disruption of excitatory neural pathways through N-methyl-D-aspartate (NMDA) (glutamate) receptor hypofunction (Coyle, 2006; Krystal et al 1994). Evidence for the role of glutamate in schizophrenia comes from many different sources. For example glutamate antagonists can cause psychotic symptoms, suggesting that schizophrenia may involve glutamate dysfunction (Kantrowitz & Javitt 2010; Coyle 2006). For example 'angel dust' or Phencyclidine (PCP), an N-methyl-D-aspartate (NMDA) antagonist, has been taken as a recreational drug particularly in the USA, and can cause positive psychotic symptoms in humans ('PCP Psychosis' has been reported). Pharmacological models employing NMDA receptor blockade by phencyclidine (PCP) and MK-801 (Cochran et al. 2003; Rujescu et al. 2006) induce changes in animal brains that have been considered to resemble those occurring in schizophrenia such as cognitive difficulties (e.g. reduced set shift ability) or reduced brain activity in prefrontal cortex (so called hypofrontality). There are also reports of altered levels of glutamate signaling pathway metabolites in cerebrospinal fluid and in post-mortem brain (Coyle, Tsai et al. 2003). Candidate genes relating to Glutamate metabolism e.g. *NRG1*, *ERBB4* and *DTNBP1* have also been found to associate with schizophrenia in some studies (Buonanno 2010). As a result of these studies and other evidence there is considerable interest in drugs that may modulate glutamatergic function in patients. Several major studies are underway including trials of LY2140023, an mGlu2/3 receptor agonist (Weinberger, 2007; Kinon et al. 2011).

Dopamine and glutamate both interact at a cortical level where glutamatergic and dopaminergic cells modulate each other: glutamatergic pyramidal cells in hippocampus and PFC are modulated by dopamine and dopaminergic firing is modulated by glutamate (see Figure 1). Perhaps in designing what individual patients require from medication, we could envisage combining different drugs needed to improve different sorts of psychopathology. For example drugs that act to improve NMDA function may improve negative, but not positive symptoms and dopaminergic antagonism may well be required to treat positive symptoms. One possible future treatment development might involve patients receiving different drug combinations to target different types of symptom domains: affective, positive, negative and cognitive (see Figure 2). In this paradigm, drugs for negative or cognitive impairment are used adjunctively with antipsychotics; indeed a number of potential cognitive enhancers are in early clinical trials at present in this way. In many ways this type of approach parallels that used in other chronic disease areas such as cancer or cardiology, where advances have been made using combinations of agents. In this way, polypharmacy could be a rational strategy, rather than viewed negatively as at present.

The search for new drugs in psychiatry will be greatly facilitated when biomarkers are available that allow patient subgroups to be identified for treatment stratification in RCTs. Biomarkers that have utility in the clinic such as genetics or EEG methods, rather than sophisticated imaging techniques such as MRI that are poorly tolerated by paranoid or anxious patients will be required. These methods used in combination with translational drug discovery paradigms rather than conventional linear drug discovery approaches (viz.

Phase 1 - 3 clinical trials) will be important drivers for drug discovery. This new approach to drug discovery combined with the search for new drug targets using the emerging understanding of the biology of schizophrenia, and the use of different drugs in combination to target different symptom domains, are likely to produce much more effective treatments in future for the schizophrenias, than those currently available.

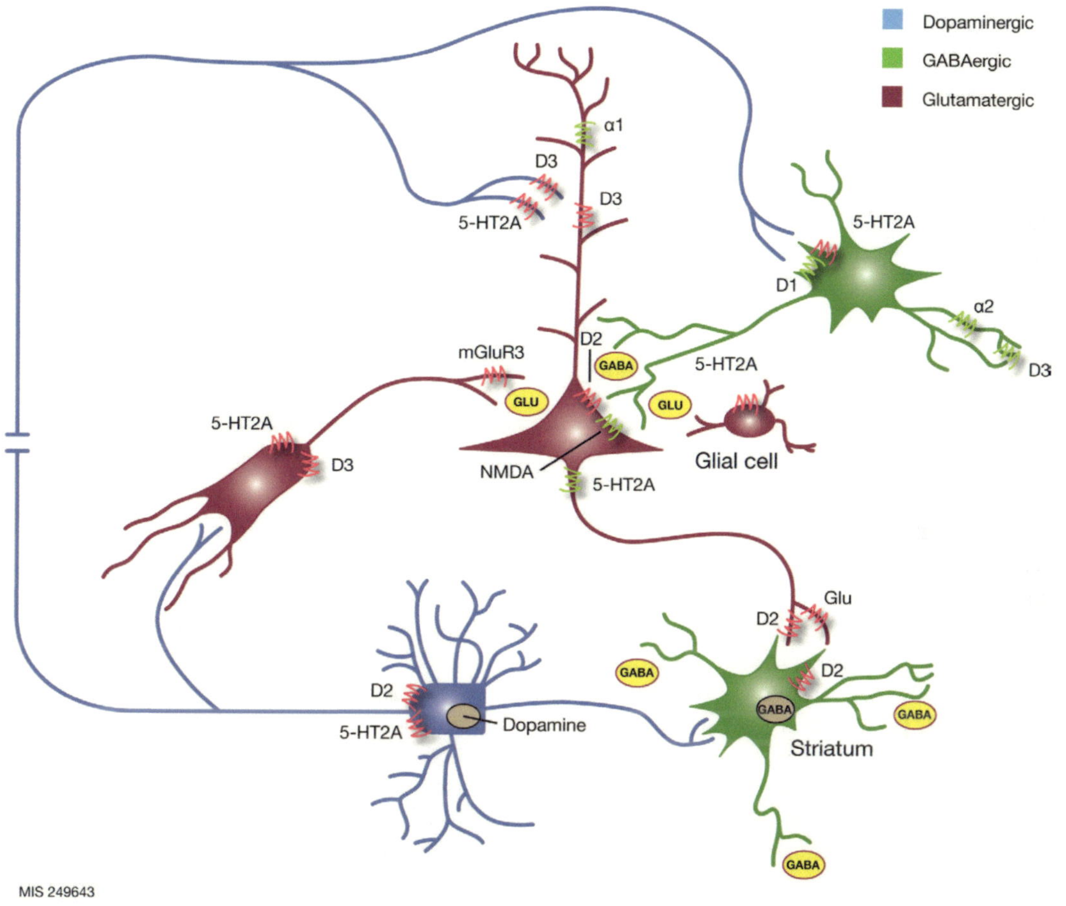

Fig. 1. Modulation of pyramidal glutamatergic neurones by GABAergic and Dopaminergic neurones. (adapted with thanks, from Nature Reviews Drug Discovery)

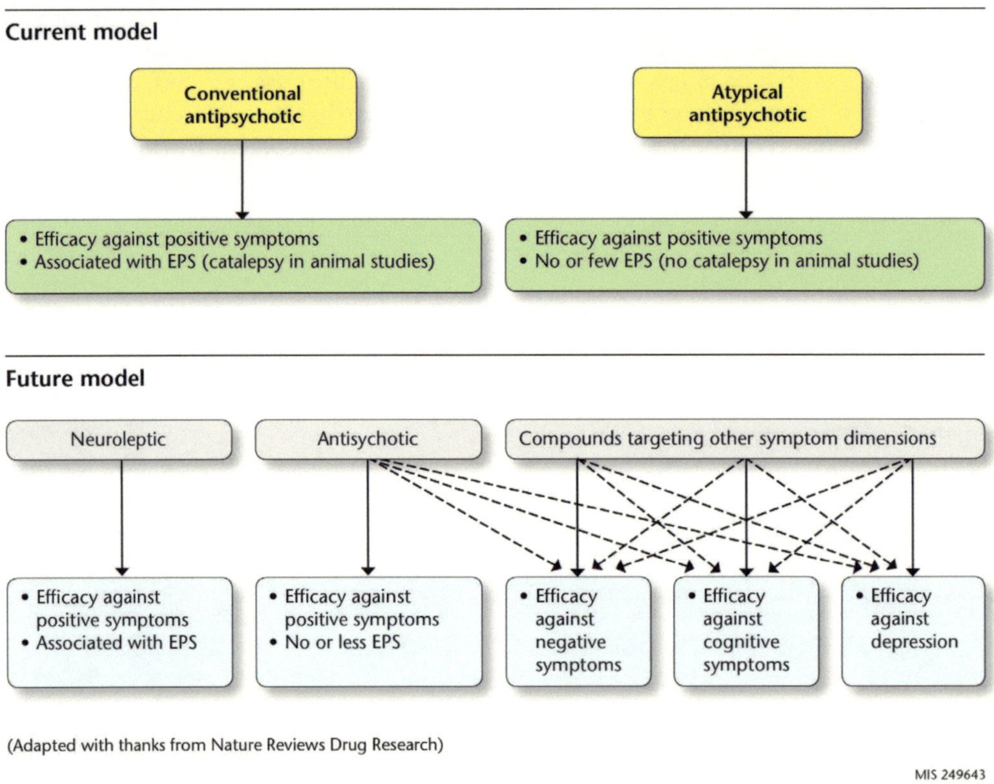

Fig. 2. Targeting symptom domains in schizophrenia: The case for rational polypharmacy.

5. Community-based care for schizophrenia

A huge change has occurred in the last few years in the way people with schizophrenia are looked after in more developed societies. Up until around the 1980s most people with serious mental health conditions were looked after in large mental hospitals (or 'institutions') many built in the Victorian era. My own hospital, Gartnavel Royal in Glasgow, dates from 1804, gaining its 'Royal' charter in 1824, and moving from the city centre to the current green field site in 1843. In the 1950s the number of resident patients peaked at over 900, almost twice the number of patients that the hospital had originally been built to accommodate. Up until the advent of what became known as 'community care', such large asylums were common throughout the UK and other countries, and existed as care communities with their own rules and mores, medical and nursing superintendents, 'therapy' of various sorts was provided such as farm work, chapels for worship, and at Gartnavel, even a golf course! Until the 1990s Glasgow, a medium sized post-industrial city, had 6 large asylums surrounding the city to accommodate people with chronic mental illness, many of whom suffered from schizophrenia. Today, with a new hospital building opened in 2008, Gartnavel Royal has only around 150 beds. Moreover most of the other asylums in Glasgow have closed completely and most patients with schizophrenia now live in the wider community. This brief example of the rise and decline of the mental hospital from Glasgow is representative of a general pattern of change that has occurred across Europe and the USA in the last two decades. While there is no doubt that one of the drivers for this change was an increased realisation of the harmful effects of institutionalisation, it is also true that financial considerations were perhaps the paramount motivation for the downsizing of mental facilities, and indeed their privatisation.

One of the countries in the vanguard of this change was Italy, where in 1978, the introduction of the Basaglia Law started a revolution in psychiatric care that concluded with the closure of the Italian state mental hospital system in 1998 (Tansella 1986). This process of reform known as *Psichiatria Democratica,* allowed for the introduction of community care and the closure of the old asylums, and was passed through the Italian Parliament with little difficulty given support across the political spectrum. Thus Italy was the first country to start a process of deinstitutionalization of mental health care and develop a community-based psychiatric system. In the UK and USA, similar developments gathered pace in the 1980s, under the leadership of Margaret Thatcher and Ronald Reagan respectively. During these changes effective and innovative service models emerged for supporting patients out with hospital and the phased closure of the psychiatric hospitals required a comprehensive, integrated community mental health service to develop. The objective of community care was an attempt to reverse the long-accepted practice of segregating the mental ill in large institutions; whether attempts to promote integration in the community have always been successful is open to question, and there is concern that many patients are now living an isolated, disconnected life in the 'community' with little regular support from psychiatric and other staff.

Most patients with schizophrenia now live in accommodation within the 'community' as demonstrated in the Scottish Schizophrenia Outcomes Study (SSOS, Hunter et al 2009). Undoubtedly there is less asylum based institutionalisation, but SSOS also demonstrated concerns about the poor quality of life and increased social isolation of the many people with schizophrenia, and the challenges for staff in supporting people in diverse settings, with pervasive positive and negative symptoms, poor psychosocial functioning, poor physical health, and vulnerability to exploitation by others. There has also been concern about the drift of many people with schizophrenia back into institutionalisation in prisons or to a life of homelessness. Individuals with comorbid personality disorders, forensic history and /or substance misuse are also a concern, and require complex, integrated models of care from motivated staff. These difficulties have been highlighted by small numbers of high profile cases where violence or homicide has occurred, sometimes due to a failure of community care supports. One well known example was the Christopher Clunis case in England (Coid, 1994), but similar failures of care have occurred in all countries.

Despite the development of community based services for people with schizophrenia and other psychotic illnesses, in-patient facilities in the UK are under considerable pressure with high rates of bed occupancy. Concern has recently been expressed by a number of groups such the Royal College of Psychiatrists in the UK and patient advocacy organisations about conditions in some in-patient facilities, which have been found to be counter therapeutic. Clearly good quality in-patient and residential facilities are essential with clear integrated care pathways and support from acute psychiatric care and rehabilitation facilities. Availability of suitable accommodation, integrated into the healthcare system, where people with schizophrenia can be supported on a regular basis and tailored to meet their needs is essential. In the UK and many other countries much of this accommodation lies within the private sector; with services sometimes having difficulty accessing patients who have failed to adhere to treatment as they become more paranoid and disorganised in their behaviour. It seems clear that while some people with schizophrenia will be able to live in their accommodation with less support, many will need a higher level of support from care workers, psychiatric nurses, and psychiatrists. Sometimes referred to as 'supported accommodation', facilities managed by a non-statutory provider such as a mental health charity, are often able to encourage socialisation, provide support, allow monitoring of mental state and behaviour, and encourage rehabilitation after the individual has left hospital. Such residential settings with mental health support workers usually have good links to local GPs, psychiatrists and the community mental health team (CMHT). Clearly in a condition where many sufferers lack insight into having mental illness, staff in the community, whether from the CMHT, primary care or mental health support workers, will all have a role to play to improve adherence to treatment plans. Twenty years ago within the asylum, the care plan for patients and the necessary communication between staff responsible for a patient's welfare appears relatively straightforward. Compare this with today's community based network of care that may involve psychiatrist and CMHT, especially the community psychiatric nurse (CPN), GP and primary care team, pharmacist, support workers from possibly several non-statutory mental health support organisations, housing associations, social work, advocacy and the legal profession. Add to this the involvement of more specialist health teams for addictions and early onset intervention, in-patient facilities at the local psychiatric unit, and as patients get older the need to involve physical health specialists and you have a highly complex network of individuals from different agencies, who need to communicate effectively and coordinate the delivery of the care plan: no mean task! Staff will increasingly need to use databases, IT networks and smart phones to meet these challenges. Schizophrenia is a long term condition, yet comprehensive long term support for the challenges patients face such as anxiety, depression, reality distortion, negative symptoms and cognitive impairments, is often less well-resourced than newer more fashionable services. For example in recent years early intervention services have been developed (Marshall & Rathbone 2011; NICE 2011), often ahead of the production of evidence of superior effectiveness for such services. In contrast the provision of adequate resources in order to develop lifelong services for people with schizophrenia that aspire to do more than treat the initial presentation, acute relapses and maintain the status quo, should be our goal.

5.1 Importance of physical healthcare

It has been estimated that people with schizophrenia have a 20% shorter life expectancy than the general population (Newman & Bland 1991), and increased vulnerability to diabetes type 2, coronary artery disease, hypertension, and emphysema. One hypothesis for such vulnerability is that the lifestyles of people with serious mental illnesses, is often associated with poor diet, obesity, lack of exercise, high rates of smoking, and use of alcohol and street drugs. Antipsychotic medication is also associated with added health risks from causally related weight gain, hyperglycaemia and the onset of diabetes, hyperlipidaemia, and abnormal findings on ECGs and cardiotoxicity. Antipsychotics have also been associated with other side effects that may affect health, including prolactin elevation, cataract formation, movement disorders, and sexual dysfunction. The significant health risks associated with schizophrenia and the medications used in its treatment, emphasise the importance of physical health monitoring in this patient population. Yet even when recognised there is evidence that patients with serious mental illness are less likely to receive standard levels of care for most diseases (De Hert et al 2011). A key priority needs to be to consider how services can be re organised to deliver better and more timely care for people with schizophrenia; while this is a challenge for inpatient care (Miller, 2011), it is an even greater challenge in relation to the majority of patients living in community settings. Solutions may vary from region to region, but will need to take account of lifestyle and local cultural factors, medication side effects, and the reluctance of, and barriers to, people with psychotic conditions contacting and using general medical services. Importantly we should also not forget the Inverse Care Law (Tudor Hart, 1971). Working as a general medical practitioner in South Wales, Tudor Hart recognised that 'the availability of good medical care tends to vary inversely with the need for it in the population served. This inverse care law operates more completely where medical care is most exposed to market forces, and less so where such exposure is reduced'. Although not written specifically about those with mental illness in mind, it would however, seem to apply no less, and given the current economic pressures in many countries for so called efficiency savings in the cost of healthcare through the use of liberalised markets, those with severe mental illness may find themselves at even greater disadvantage than at present. An important next step in the management of physical health in this population will be to improve awareness and training in those doctors, including psychiatrists, who already care for the mentally ill, and to encourage them to follow guidelines for standardizing investigations, assessments and care given to mental health patients. Recommendations include taking regular measurements of patients' weight and BMI, monitoring blood pressure, checking glucose levels and carefully evaluating their medication history. Smoking is more prevalent in people with schizophrenia than comparisons with the general population, but encouragingly there has been some success in the use of specialist services for smoking cessation help.

5.2 Psychosocial interventions

It is beyond the scope of this chapter to review in detail the increasing trend to employ psychosocial adjunctive methods in the treatment plan for people with schizophrenia. Lack of insight and poor adherence to treatment often present formidable challenges to those involved in care, as well as blocking roads to recovery. NICE (2011) has recommended that family intervention should be offered to all individuals diagnosed with schizophrenia that are in close contact with, or live with, family members and should be considered a priority where there are persistent symptoms or a high risk of relapse. Family intervention should include communication skills, problem solving and psycho-education. Psycho-educational approaches have been developed to increase patients' knowledge about, and insight into, their illness and treatment. A recent Cochrane review (Xia et al 2011) compared the efficacy of psycho-education added to standard care with that of standard care alone, and the meta-analysis showed a significant reduction of relapse or readmission rates. As the authors admit however there is a scarcity of good quality studies of adequate power, and difficulties in combining studies with different definitions of what is meant by psycho-education. A recent review of the evidence for psycho-educational interventions to improve adherence to antipsychotic medication, behavioural interventions, or compliance therapy, concluded that the jury is still out due to due to a paucity of good quality evidence (Barry et al 2012).

Although Cognitive Behavioural Therapy (CBT) was first reported as a possible therapy for people with schizophrenia in 1952, it was not recommended as a routine treatment until 2009. Research on positive symptoms has led to the hypothesis that there are specific cognitive biases affecting reasoning, attribution style and impaired self-worth (e.g. see Garety and Freeman, 1999). This led to the development of models and interventions for positive symptoms based on Cognitive Behavioural Therapy (e.g. Kuipers et al 2006 and Moritz &

Woodward, 2007). Over the last few years modified CBT for psychosis (or CBTp) has been developed. This is described as a structured and collaborative therapeutic approach, which purports to be a discrete psychological intervention. CBTp aims to make explicit connections between thinking, emotions, physiology and behaviour with respect to current or past problems. CBTp also seeks to achieve systemic change through the re-evaluation of perceptions, beliefs or reasoning hypothesised to cause and maintain psychiatric symptoms and psychological problems. The aim of CBTp seems overly ambitious for most patients, but may help for the individual make sense of their psychotic experiences, and reduce the associated distress and impact on functioning. Targeted outcomes, though not always achieved, include symptom reduction (positive or negative symptoms and general symptoms including mood), relapse reduction, enhancement of social functioning, development of insight, amelioration of distress, and the promotion of recovery. Although there is support for CBTp and in England it is recommended by NICE (2011), other evidence is more equivocal such as the Cochrane Review in 2011 which concludes that Trial-based evidence suggests no clear and convincing advantage for cognitive behavioural therapy over other and sometimes much less sophisticated therapies for people with schizophrenia (Jones et al 2011).

The effectiveness of available interventions for negative symptoms is far from satisfactory: Cognitive-behavioral therapy (CBTp) shows some impact on negative symptoms but the effect sizes are small (Wykes et al 2008). Even psychosocial approaches specifically developed to reduce negative symptoms have failed to produce convincing effects.

6. Rehabilitation, recovery and recovery-based services

Perhaps surprisingly, the advent of the asylums in the late 18th century was associated with therapeutic optimism, as 'moral treatment' for the mentally unwell was advocated. Such treatment emphasized an optimistic approach, physical activity, minimal coercion and comfortable, healthy environments for people with serious mental health problems and recovery was defined as the abatement of symptoms (Tuke, 1813). However by the beginning of the 20th century, the asylums were overcrowded, a situation which lasted well into the 1990s and the early optimism gave way to different approaches which emphasised containment, loss of more personalised approaches and the classification of mental disorders by Kraepelin and Bleuler tended to stress the chronic and often progressive course in people diagnosed with schizophrenia. Throughout the last 50 years the use of neuroleptic medication - the major tranquilisers, soon rebranded as 'antipsychotics' - has been recognised to help the abatement of positive symptoms. However in the late 20th century, a different notion of what recovery might mean, re-entered the mental health arena that had echoes back to the optimism of the early asylum era. The developments in psychiatric rehabilitation and deinstitutionalisation, as well the developing service user/survivor

movement gave the term recovery new meanings in the late 1980s and the 1990s. Unlike the traditional clinical understanding of recovery, focussing on the abatement of symptoms, this new use of 'recovery' did not necessarily equate with abatement of symptoms but instead emphasised a renewed sense of self and encouragement for a return to a more self-directed meaningful life (Mental Health Commission of New Zealand, 2011). This distinction between clinical recovery and personal recovery has not always been well understood by mental health practitioners although there is increasing evidence that practitioners are now increasingly using the principles of recovery in their work (Lieberman et al 2008; Davidson et al 2006).

Lieberman attempted a synthesis between the different perspectives, arguing that clinical neuroscience (psychiatric practice) and the newer meanings of recovery, as defined by the advocacy movement were complementary and not mutually exclusive or competing (Lieberman et al 2008). However it should be recognised that some proponents of the 'recovery movement', view most mainstream psychiatric services as emphasising an approach where 'the assessment of personal deficits' is an important element. This would include rehabilitation services, which while apparently more optimistic and 'recovery-focused', share with acute mental health services the same philosophy namely that treatment should follow assessment of 'deficits' (symptoms, issues, impairments etc.). The service user/survivor movement on the other hand, is based on the notion of self-determination and developing personal strengths and has been influenced by social models of disability which assert that it is society that disables, not the impairments of individuals (Oliver, 1990). Consequently some of the recovery literature coming out of the user/survivor movement may be more likely to question the basic tenets of the mental health system such as the concept of mental illness itself, or the need for compulsory treatment, or the process of assessing individuals' needs or difficulties. Unfortunately there is sometimes an impression that some proponents of the recovery movement are not only challenging, but antagonistic towards the views and expertise of mental health professionals who are sometimes caricatured as being stuck in a traditional mind set, cataloguing deficits and beholden to medicalised models of mental health (Slade, 2009). In is not an overstatement to say that developing interventions and strategies to improve mental health will clearly benefit from all interested parties sharing ideas, learning from one another and working together in respectful manner. Interestingly survivor literature on recovery often tends to focus on the deficits external to the individual with the diagnosis, for example in support services or housing in wider society, more than in the individual themselves. In the author's experience rehabilitation team professionals often echo similar views in their frustration to help people find meaning in their lives: at Gartnavel Royal Hospital the legacy of Dr RD Laing is never far from one's mind.

Encouragingly there does appear to be a developing shared understanding of the importance of personal recovery within rehabilitation, and other mental health professionals. One simple yet powerful technique promoted in recovery is supporting an individual to make sense of what has happened in their life; such life stories can not only help someone add meaning to their life, and move forward, but may also help professionals and carers to understand their journey (Scotti 2009). The Scottish Recovery Network (SRN) (http://www.scottishrecovery.net) has promoted this idea in its Narrative Research Project which has provided support for people to tell their stories. In Table 3, the Key Themes of Recovery from the SRN are described in more detail including: recovery as a journey; hope, optimism and strengths; more than recovery from illness; control, choice, and inclusion; self-management; finding meaning and purpose; relationships.

Recovery as a journey

The recovery journey can have ups and downs and some people describe being *in recovery* rather than recovered to reflect this.

Hope, optimism and strengths

Hope is widely acknowledged as key to recovery. There can be no change without the belief that a better life is both possible and attainable. One way to realise a more hopeful approach is to find ways to focus on strengths.

More than recovery from illness

Some people describe being in recovery while still experiencing symptoms. For some it is about recovering a life and *identity* beyond the experience of mental ill health.

Control, choice and inclusion

Taking control can be hard but many people describe how it important it is to find a way to take an active and responsible role in their own recovery. Control is supported by the inclusion of people with experience of mental health issues in their communities. It is reduced by the experience of *exclusion, stigma* and *discrimination*.

Self-management

One way to gain more control over recovery is to develop and use self-management techniques. One such self-management tool which Scottish Recovery Network promotes is the Wellness Recovery Action Plan.

Finding meaning and purpose

We all find meaning in very different ways. Some people may find spirituality important, while others may find meaning through employment or the development of stronger interpersonal or community links. Many people describe the importance of feeling valued and of *contributing* as active members of a community.

Relationships

Supportive relationships based on belief, trust and shared humanity help promote recovery.

Table 3. Key Themes of Recovery*
*Reprinted with thanks from the Scottish Recovery Network:
http://www.scottishrecovery.net/

While recovery is a unique and individual experience it is possible to identify key themes and ideas in relation to the experience. The above list, while not exhaustive, highlights some of the most commonly identified elements.

Psychiatric rehabilitation had its origins in the programme of asylum closures in the 1980s and 90s with the aim of helping community integration and promotion of independence of individuals with mental health problems. But where then does psychiatric rehabilitation stand today, following deinstitutionalisation and the influence of the recovery movement? Today the focus of much of the work within many rehabilitation services in the UK is with individuals who have not progressed within acute admission wards and are unable to be discharged, because of a complex interplay of factors between the individual and their environment. Often rehabilitation teams, comprising psychiatrists, social workers, nurses, psychologists and occupational therapists and other mental health professionals, work to reduce functional impairments and the intensity of symptoms using a variety of approaches, combining pharmacological treatment, independent living and social skills training, psychological support to individuals and their families, housing, and access to meaningful activities. The ethos of the rehabilitation team is to work collaboratively in order to empower people to find their way forward and live a meaningful life. Clearly the recovery movement has influenced, and continues to influence the development of rehabilitation (and other) services, some of which are now being rebranded as 'supported recovery services'. The Scottish Recovery Network has produced a web-based tool (Scottish Recovery Indicator, SRI) that has been designed to help mental health services facilitate change in practice and promote a more recovery orientated service. Some NHS services in Scotland are using to the SRI tool to help service providers assess the extent to which their services are 'recovery focussed'. Most such initiatives are management, rather than professionally, driven, but do usefully highlight issues in relation to inclusion, rights, equalities and diversity. Personal recovery approaches have become central to mental health policy in many English-speaking countries. A comparative analysis of policy direction in seven countries (New Zealand, Australia, Canada, England, Scotland, USA and Italy) notes a good deal of convergence in their priorities. It is instructive to list these priorities as they give an important outline of the shape of services in many modern psychiatric care systems and also emphasise how influential the recovery movement has been. The following themes occur throughout the seven services: promotion of wellbeing and anti-discrimination; improving access and enhancing range of services; ensuring an adequate, competent and skilled workforce; focusing on service user participation, responsiveness and recovery; integrating / linking health and social sectors; promoting evidence-based, measurable and accountable responses; wellbeing promotion and prevention; early intervention and anti-discrimination; 'holistic' responses for people with mental illness including talking therapies, drug therapies, peer support, recovery education, support in crisis, support in housing, support in education and employment, and advocacy (Compagni, Adams & Daniels, 2006).

7. Future directions

As we consider the centenary of Bleuler's influential monograph and the introduction of the term 'schizophrenia', it is timely to ask how much progress has been made in understanding the pathogenesis of schizophrenia and the development of effective treatments. As will be clear from this chapter, despite the considerable advances in neuroscience, there is still some way to go in understanding the neuroscience of schizophrenia. We still have much to learn about what changes in brain structure and function occur and why. Despite the advances in genetics in the last few years, what we know is that schizophrenia probably involves multiple genetic markers - perhaps more than 1000 genes - involved in establishing and maintaining a complex network of molecular relationships within the brain. We still have much to understand about gene interactions, gene expression and how environmental effects, such as psycho-social stressors and trauma, may affect gene expression and cell function. We are also beginning to appreciate that psycho-social factors may also impact on brain structure and function via genetic and non-genetic mechanisms, particularly at vulnerable times in development, but how this occurs is poorly understood despite interesting work in animal models. It seems clear however, that only from an understanding of the biology of pathogenesis will more coherent and better treatments eventually emerge. It is very concerning recently that a number of major pharmaceutical companies have decided to move out of CNS research, and in particular schizophrenia research, due to the scale of current challenges, including the lack of good drug targets, and lack of effective techniques and methods for diagnosing and/or stratifying patient populations, and monitoring response. There is an urgent need to make progress on the development of biomarkers that have utility in ordinary clinical settings: MRI or SPECT/PET scanning will be useful research tools in specialised settings but none of these imaging methods will support the sort of biomarkers we require: low cost, easily accessible, and available in clinics that patients are comfortable about visiting. Genetic and EEG methods look the most promising in this regards with data being sent electronically to expert centres for fast reporting back to clinicians. This sort of telemedicine approach is likely to develop first in memory clinics for the assessment of Alzheimer's disease, but will probably then move to schizophrenia, if biomarkers are available.

These advances are likely to be some way off but there are approaches we could introduce now to begin to develop a more personalized medicine approach in schizophrenia. We have discussed above that schizophrenia needs to be seen as a long term condition and a more integrated care pathway developed that recognises this. Many guidelines for schizophrenia appear to be little more than a list of short term interventions advocated on the basis of a less than adequate evidence base, where conflicts of interest of authors are seldom transparent. In my view guidelines need to utilize the framework of the patient's timeline, and in this way the challenges of middle and late stage illness may receive the attention they merit. It is still quite puzzling and unhelpful that most psychiatrists do not use any sytematic set of standardized assessments. Symptoms and functionality are reported in narrative, subjective form, without the use of any form of adjunctive standardised assessment. It is diificult to understand why this has occurred, given the absence of any biomarkers in psychiatry. In my view mental health specialists, but particularly psychiatrists need to agree on a menu of measures in order to standardise the assessment of positive, negative, cognitive and psycho-social functioning in schizophrenia. While Bleuler is to be praised for his detailed clinical descriptions, the quality of which appear absent from many case notes today, 100 years later we should be moving to a system of more standardized assessment in order to augment narrative descriptions using available reliable and valid instruments. These measures could usefully help clinicians assess, in a more individulaised way, which areas of need are a priority for individual patients, and would facillitate better mapping of progress and assessment of outcome. Although such methods have been embraced by psychologists and even nurses within mental health, and by physicians in other specialties (e.g. Apgar Scores by paediatriacians: Casey et al 2001; Glasgow Coma Scale by neurologists: Matis & Birbilis 2008), psychiatrists, at least in most of the UK, but probably more widely, seem uniquely resistant to this development. Gilbody et al (2002) reported a survey of the use of outcome measures in psychiatric practice in the UK involving 500 consultant psychiatrists practising in the NHS and reported that only 6.5% of clinicians treating patients with schizophrenia routinely used standardised measures to assess clinical changes over time. At a recent focus group on this issue (personal communication), this resistance was still evident; some of the views noted included: 'standardized measures are appropriate for research but not clinical practice'; 'divides a continuously fluctuating process into arbitrary categories'; 'assessments have poor psychometric properties: validity, reliability and sensitivity to change'; 'detracts from therapeutic relationship'. It is interesting that DSM-5 may well embrace this type of dimensional approach within broad diagnostic categories. Such an approach could begin to help develop and tailor pharmacological and psychological interventions for individual patients. For example, packages of care could be planned to meet an individual's needs for control of positive, affective or negative symptoms, and cognitive impairments. Personalised medicine though is not just about assessments and tailoring interventions, it is also about listening to patients (and their carers) and working with them to promote clinical and personal recovery.

There is no doubt that the social and institutional reforms in many developed countries, with emphasis on human rights, dignity, and attempts (as yet not too successful) to reduce stigma have been important steps forward. The change from institutionalised care in large isolated asylums, to community based care using smaller scale modern facilities, has been important. While I have discussed the limitations of antipsychotic medication, there is no doubt that the availability of such medication has made an important contribution to the management of acute episodes and prevention of relapse. The philosophical approach of personal recovery is becoming better accepted by mental health professionals and has been incorporated into the care offered to many patients by many services. As we understand better the biology of schizophrenia, rational opportunities to develop more effective and less toxic treatments will follow. However it is likely that more effective psychological interventions such as cognitive remediation (McGurk et al 2007; Wykes & Spaulding 2011) will also become important and we will be clearer about what constitutes the key elements of successful talking treatments. It is interesting that such therapies appear to be evolving from quite a narrow CBT focus to talking therapies that involve a broader scope that embraces the principles of personal recovery.

So what's next for schizophrenia as the century unfolds? The brain is by far the most complex organ and organisation in the known world. Comparisons with computers or the internet are rather facile, and probably unhelpful. Our understanding of neuroscience and specifically of the brain will continue to progress given adequate human and economic resources, although current reductionist approaches may have limitations in understanding the complexity involved. It is likely that advances from other scientific disciplines such as physics, mathematics, genetics and molecular biology will help to provide new insights into how psychiatric disturbance is caused and maintained. Such insights may help identify new potential treatments; however it is likely that knowledge from areas as yet not envisioned or conceptualised may provide a paradigm shift in our thinking about psychiatric illness and schizophrenia that hopefully will herald much more progress in the 21st century, than the modest progress we have seen in the last since Bleuler.

8. References

Aleman A, Kahn RS, Selten JP (2003). Sex differences in the risk of schizophrenia. Evidence from meta-analysis. Archives General Psychiatry 60, 565–571.

Barry S, Gaughan T & Hunter R (2012). Schizophrenia. BMJ Clinical Evidence (in press).

Bleuler E (1911). Dementia praecox oder die Gruppe der Schizophrenien. Leipzig, Germany: Deuticke; 1911.

Bleuler E (1911). Dementia Praecox or the Group of Schizophrenias. Zinkin J, trans. New York, NY: International University Press; 1950

Bleuler E (1911). Die Psychoanalyse Freuds. Verteidigung und kritische bemerkungen. Jahrbuch fu¨r Psychoanalytische und Psychopathologische Forschungen. 2, 1–110.

Buchanan RW, David M, Goff G et al (2005). A summary of the FDA-NIMH-MATRICS workshop on clinical trial design for neurocognitive drugs for schizophrenia. Schizophrenia Bulletin 31, 1-15

Buonanno (2010). The neuregulin signaling pathway and schizophrenia: from genes to synapses and neural circuits. Brain Res Bull. 83:122–131.

Coid JW (1994). The Christopher Clunis Enquiry. Psychiatric Bulletin, 18:449-452

Casey BM, McIntyre D & Leveno K (2001). The continuing value of the Apgar score for the assessment of newborn infants. New England Journal of Medicine 344, 467-71.

Cochran, SM et al. Induction of metabolic hypofunction and neurochemical deficits after chronic intermittent exposure to phencyclidine: differential modulation by antipsychotic drugs. Neuropsychopharmacology 28, 265-275 (2003).

Collins PY, Patel V, Joestl SS, March D, Insel TR et al (2011). Grand challenges in global mental health. Nature 475, 27-30.

Compagni, A., Adams, N. & Daniels, A. (2006). International pathways to mental health system transformation: Strategies and challenges. Sacramento: California Institute for Mental Health. http://www.cimh.org/Services/Special-Projects/International-Pathways.aspx.

Coyle, J T, Tsai, G & Goff, D (2003). Converging evidence of NMDA receptor hypofunction in the pathophysiology of schizophrenia. Annals of the New York Academy of Sciences, 1003: 318–327.

Coyle JT (2006). Glutamate and Schizophrenia: Beyond the Dopamine Hypothesis. Cellular and Molecular Neurobiology, 26, 365-383.

Cuthbert BN, and Insel TR (2010). Toward new approaches to psychotic disorders: the NIMH research domain criteria project. Schizophr Bull 2010; 36: 1061-1062.

Davidson, L., O'Connell, M., Tondora, J., Styron, T. & Kangas, K. (2006). The top ten concerns about recovery encountered in mental health system transformation. Psychiatric Services, 57, 640–645.

De Hert M, Correll CU, Bobes J, Cetkovich-bakmas M, et al (2011). Physical illness in patients with severe mental disorders: 1. Prevalence, impact of medication and disparities in health care. World Psychiatry 10, 52-77.

Delay J, Deniker P, Harl JM (1952). Utilisation en thérapeutique d'une phénothiazine d'action centrale selective. Annales Médico-psychologiques 110, 112–7.

European Psychiatry http://www.ncbi.nlm.nih.gov/pubmed/21602034

Garety P, and Freeman D (1999). Cognitive approaches to delusions: a critical review of theories and evidence. British Journal of Clinical Psychology 38: 113-154.

Gilbody S et al (2002). Why do UK psychiatrists not use outcome measures? British Journal of Psychiatry 180:101–103.

Green MF (1996). What are the functional consequences of neurocognitive deficits in schizophrenia? American J Psychiatry, 153, 321–330.

Harvey P, Koren D, Reichenberg A et al (2006). Negative symptoms and cognitive deficits: what is the nature of their relationship? Schizophrenia Bulletin 32, 250-258.

Huffaker SJ, Chen J, Nicodemus KK, et al (2009). A primate-specific, brain isoform of KCNH2 affects cortical physiology, cognition, neuronal repolarization and risk of schizophrenia. Nature Medicine , 15, 509-518.

Hunter R & Barry S (2011a). Negative symptoms and psychosocial functioning in EGOFORS: neglected but important targets for treatment. European Psychiatry http://www.ncbi.nlm.nih.gov/pubmed/21602034

Hunter R, Barry, S & Gaughan T (2012). Schizophrenia. BMJ Clinical Evidence (in press).

Hunter R, Cameron R & Norrie J (2009). Using patient-reported outcomes in schizophrenia: The Scottish Schizophrenia Outcomes Study. Psychiatric Services 60, 2, 240 - 245.

Jablensky A, Sartorius N, Ernberg G, et al. (1992). Schizophrenia: manifestations, incidence and course in different cultures. A World Health Organization ten-country study. Psychol Med Monogr Suppl 20:1–97.

Johnstone EC (1993). Schizophrenia: problems in clinical practice. Lancet 341:536–538

Jones C, Hacker D, Meadenac I, Irving CB (2011). Cognitive behaviour therapy versus other psychosocial treatments for schizophrenia. Cochrane Database of Systematic Reviews 2011, Issue 4. Art. No.: CD000524. DOI: 10.1002/14651858.CD000524.pub3.

Kane JM, Honigfeld G, Singer J, et al. (1988). Clozapine for the treatment-resistant schizophrenic. Archives General Psychiatry, 45, 789–796.

Kantrowitz JT & Javitt DC (2010). N-methyl-d-aspartate (NMDA) receptor dysfunction or dysregulation: The final common pathway on the road to schizophrenia? Brain Research Bulletin 83, 108-21.

Kinon BJ, Zhang L, Millen BA, et al (2011). A multicenter, inpatient, phase 2, double-blind, placebo controlled dose-ranging study of LY2140023 monohydrate in patients with DSM-IV schizophrenia. Journal of Clinical Psychopharmacology, 31: 349–55.

Kirkpatrick B, Fenton WS, Carpenter WT, Marder SR (2006). The NIMH-MATRICS consensus statement on negative symptoms. Schizophr Bull, 32, 214-219.

Kraepelin E (1919). Dementia praecox and paraphrenia. Translated by Barclay RM. New York: RE Krieger; 1971.

Krystal, JH, Karper LP, Seibyl,JP, Freeman GK, Delaney R, Bremner JD, Heninger GR, Bowers MB & Charney,DS (1994). Subanesthetic Effects of the Non-competitive NMDA Antagonist Ketamine, in Humans. Archives General Psychiatry 51, 199-214.

Kuipers E, Garety P, Fowler D, Freeman D, Dunn G, and Bebbington P (2006). Cognitive, emotional, and social processes in psychosis: refining cognitive behavioral therapy for persistent positive symptoms. Schizophrenia Bulletin 32, 24-31.

Laughren T & Levin R (2011) Food and Drug Administration Commentary on methodological issues in negative symptom trials. Schizophrenia Bulletin 37, 255-256.

Leucht S, Hierla S, Kissling W, Dold M, Davis JM (2011). Putting the efficacy of psychiatric and general medicine medication in perspective: A review of meta-analyses. British Journal Psychiatry. In Press.

Lieberman JA, Drake RE, Sederer LI, Belger A, Keefe R, Perkins D, Stroup S (2008). Science and Recovery in schizophrenia. Psychiatric Services 59:487-496.

Mäkinen J, Miettunen M, Isohanni & Koponen H (2008). Negative symptoms in schizophrenia - a review. Nordic Journal of Psychiatry, 62, 334-341.

Marshall M, Rathbone J (2011). Early intervention for psychosis. Cochrane Database of Systematic Reviews 2011, Issue 6. Marder R, Essock SM, Miller, AL et al (2004). Physical Health Monitoring of Patients with Schizophrenia. American Journal of Psychiatry 161:1334–1349.

Matis & Birbilis (2008). Glasgow Coma Scale. Acta Neurol Belg 108:75–89.

McGrath JJ (2006). Variations in the incidence of schizophrenia: data versus dogma. Schizophrenia Bulletin. 32, 195–197.

McGurk S, Twamley EW, Sitzer DI, McHugi GJ, Mueser KT (2007). A meta-analysis of cognitive remediation in schizophrenia. American J Psychiatry 164, 1791-1802.

Mental Health Commission of New Zealand (2011). Recovery meanings and measures. http://www.mhc.govt.nz

Miller BJ (2011). Hospital admission for schizophrenia and bipolar disorder. British Medical Journal 343, 596-7.

Moritz S, Woodward TS (2007). Metacognitive training in schizophrenia: from basic research to knowledge translation and intervention. . Current Opinion in Psychiatry 20, 619–625.

Newman SC, Bland RC (1991). Mortality in a cohort of patients with schizophrenia: a record linkage study. Canadian J Psychiatry 36, 239–245.

NICE (2011). Schizophrenia: Core interventions in the treatment and management of schizophrenia in primary and secondary care (update) 2011. National Clinical Practice Guideline Number 82, National Collaborating Centre for Mental Health. 2009, National Institute for Health and Clinical Excellence: London, UK.

Oliver, M (1990). The politics of disablement. London: MacMillan.

Picchioni MM, Murray RM. Schizophrenia (2007). British Medical Journal 335, 91–95.

Purcell, S.M., Wray, N.R., Stone, J.L., Visscher, P.M., O'Donovan, M.C., Sullivan, P.F. and Sklar, P. (2009) Common polygenic variation contributes to risk of schizophrenia and bipolar disorder. Nature, 460, 748-52.

Rujescu D, Bender A et al (2006). A pharmacological model for psychosis based on N-methyl-D-aspartate receptor hypofunction: molecular, cellular, functional and behavioral abnormalities. Biol Psychiatry 59, 721-9

Scotti, P (2009). Recovery as Discovery. Schizophrenia Bulletin 35, 844–846.

Scottish Association for Mental Health (SAMH, 2007). The social and economic costs of mental health problems in Scotland. Sainsbury Centre for Mental Health, UK.

Shi, J., Levinson, D.F., Duan, J., Sanders, A.R., Zheng, Y., Pe'er, I., Dudbridge, F., Holmans, P.A., Whittemore, A.S., Mowry, B.J. et al. (2009). Common variants on chromosome 6p22.1 are associated with schizophrenia. Nature, 460, 753-7.

Slade, M. (2009). Personal recovery and mental illness: A guide for mental health professionals. New York: Cambridge University Press.

Stefansson, H., Ophoff, R.A., Steinberg, S., Andreassen, O.A., Cichon, S., Rujescu, D., Werge, T., Pietilainen, O.P., Mors, O., Mortensen, P.B. et al. (2009).

Sullivan PF, Kendler KS & Neal MC (2003). Schizophrenia as a Complex Trait. Evidence From a Meta-analysis of Twin Studies. Arch Gen Psychiatry 60, 1187-1192.

Tamminga CA & Holcomb HH (2005). Phenotype of schizophrenia: a review and formulation. Molecular Psychiatry 10, 27–39.

Tansella M. (1986). Community psychiatry without mental hospitals: the Italian experience: a review. Journal of the Royal Society of Medicine 79, 664–669.

Tudor Hart, J (1971). The inverse care law. The Lancet 297, 405-412.

Tuke, S. (1813) Description of the retreat. London: Process Press (1996).

Van Rossum, JM (1966). The significance of dopamine-receptor blockade for the mechanism of action of neuroleptic drugs. Archives Internationales de Pharmacodynamie et de Therapie 160, 492-4.

Weinberger, D (2007). Schizophrenia drug says goodbye to dopamine. Nature Medicine 13, 1018.

World Health Organization (WHO, 2008). The Global Burden of Disease; 2004 Update.

Wykes T & Spaulding WD (2011). Thinking about the future cognitive remediation therapy - what works and could we do better? Schizophrenia Bulletin, 37 suppl. 2, S80–S90.

Wykes T, Steel C, Everitt B, Tarrier N (2008). Cognitive behavior therapy for schizophrenia: effect sizes, clinical models, and methodological rigor. Schizophrenia Bulletin 34, 523-537.

Xia J, Merinder LB, Belgamwar MR (2011). Psychoeducation for schizophrenia. Cochrane Library of Systematic Reviews, November 2011.

2

Family Caregivers of People with Schizophrenia in East Asian Countries

Setsuko Hanzawa
Jichi Medical University
Japan

1. Introduction

Public endorsement of mental illness stigma impacts many people. People with mental illness, their families, service providers, and the general public are all groups of special importance when considering stigma. The harm that public stigma causes people who are labeled mentally ill is perhaps of the greatest concern. Their family members and friends are also impacted by public stigma (Phelan et al., 1998). It has been extensively documented that caregivers of persons who have serious and persistent mental disorders must successfully cope with many challenging problems in order to provide good care.

This chapter was written to help European and American people understand the unique aspects of family caregivers' recognition and attitude toward people with schizophrenia in Japan and Korea, East Asian countries. These aspects are based on Confucian ideas and the tradition of providing care for dependents. We discuss the need for support for family caregivers, derived from our family-related studies. We also discuss the current issues of mental health infrastructure and compulsory community treatment, instead of inpatient facilities, for persons with chronic schizophrenia and their family caregivers.

2. A long-term hospitalization system in Japan and Korea

As is known worldwide, Japan formerly had a long-term hospitalization system and a hospital detention policy that involuntarily admitted people with mental diseases to psychiatric hospitals. Many inpatient psychiatric facilities exist today. For example, in 2005, the number of psychiatric beds per 10,000 populations was 28 in Japan, and 14 in South Korea (World Health Organization [WHO], 2005). Compared to South Korea, Japan has higher rate of total psychiatric beds in mental hospitals, general hospitals, and other settings.

South Korea has the higher rate of psychiatric beds in other settings, such as unrecognized "houses of prayer" than Japan. The number of Japanese psychiatric beds continued to be over 25 per 10,000 populations from 1994 to 2005. On the other hand, the number of South Korean psychiatric beds saw a steady increase from 2.8 to 13.8 during the same period. In South Korea, the formulation of the Mental Health Act of 1995 led many private mental asylums to be changed into mental hospitals. Different psychosocial programs have been developed for rehabilitation, open wards are slowly developing in mental hospitals, and unrecognized "houses of prayer" have been closed.

In Japan and South Korea, both custodial care in mental hospitals and prolonged inappropriate stays of patients persist, primarily due to a lack of adequate staff to care for patients in the community. The length of an inpatient stay is still very long and a great deal of stigma still remains against mental disorders and patients.

2.1 Two kinds of involuntary hospitalization

Interestingly, in Japan and Korea, two forms of "Involuntary Hospitalization" are allowed by the current mental health laws. In Japan, the law is the Law Related to Mental Health and Welfare of the Person with Mental Disorder. One form is "Involuntary Hospitalization", which is intended for the treatment and care for individuals deemed likely to hurt themselves or others because of mental disorder based upon abnormal behavior and other circumstances. Another form is "Hospitalization for Medical Care and Protection", which is intended for the treatment and care of individuals who are judged to be mentally disordered based upon examination by a designated physician and who need hospitalization for medical care and protection. "Hospitalization for Medical Care and Protection" requires the family's consent instead of the patient's consent, and it has been allowed since 1950 by the Mental Hygiene Law. Furthermore, in these countries, family caregivers are obligated to do the following: (1) protect the person with a mental disorder to ensure treatment and the protection of his or her proprietary interests, (2) cooperate with the physician to ensure that the person with the mental disorder is correctly diagnosed, and (3) comply with the physician's instructions to ensure medical care for the person with the mental disorder. Therefore, family members of people with mental disorders have experienced guilt related to "involuntary hospitalization" for many years. Additionally, the family member with the mental illness often blames their family members for giving consent. Involuntary psychiatric hospitalization has led to complex family relationships in Japan, especially because patients have little insight into the seriousness of the illness during the acute delusional stage of schizophrenia and later forget these situations.

2.1.1 Compulsory admission and compulsory community treatment

The mental health laws dictate the family's obligation to ensure treatment and medical care for the patient. The mental health laws explain that the compulsory admission requires the family's consent, rather than the patient's consent. However, the laws do not dictate professional compulsory community treatment in Japan and South Korea.

Pervasive negative attitudes and discriminatory treatment towards people with mental illness are well documented in Northeast Asian countries and in Chinese societies. The particular manifestations of the stigma associated with schizophrenia are shaped by cultural meanings based on Confucianism. These cultural meanings are reflected in severe cultural-specific expressions of stigma in Chinese societies (Yang, 2007). In contrast to the political personhood of the West, in which a Westerner considers family as a volitional option, the familial personhood of the East stands on the foundation of a family with each individual understanding that "filial piety is one of the roots of humanity" (Lee, 2009). Both Japan and

South Korea are located in East Asia and have cultures based on Confucian ideas and the tradition of providing care for dependents.

In contrast, in Taiwan of one of East Asian countries, a 2010 Taiwanese pilot program is implementing compulsory community treatment to reduce the "revolving door phenomenon". This pilot program theoretically serves as a substitute for compulsory admission, discharge planning or condition discharge, and relapse prevention. According to the 2007 Mental Health Act, the process begins when severely mentally ill patients do not comply with medical orders and thus are living in unstable conditions or are feared to jeopardize their daily function. In order to participate in the pilot program, the severely mentally ill patient's community treatment must have been recommended by a board certified psychiatrist, and the patient must have refused or failed to give consent. If necessary, policemen and firefighters may assist by completing the above measures under appropriate requests. Non-government organizations (NGOs) approved by the government may monitor the compulsory community treatment.

2.1.2 Regional and socio-cultural differences in East Asia

Recently, factors influencing the extent of caregiver burden have attracted attention. Patient variables, caregiver characteristics, and regional differences have been identified as predictors of caregiver burden (Roick et al., 2006). Caregiver burden can also reflect regional differences in patients' socio-economic situations and family support in European countries (Magliano et al., 2002) and in the provision of rehabilitative interventions for patients (Magliano et al., 2001). Roick and colleagues reported that the burden placed on family members of people with schizophrenia may be influenced not only by patient and caregiver characteristics but also by national differences in the provision of mental health care services (Roick et al., 2007). This assumption was evaluated by comparing caregivers in Germany and Britain, two northern European countries that differ appreciably in their provision of mental health services. Even after controlling for patient and caregiver characteristics, British caregivers reported a significantly higher level of burden than did German caregivers (Roick et al., 2007). In another comparison study, a higher burden was observed in Italy and Britain as compared to the Netherlands, Spain and Denmark. These differences were attributed to differences in the provision of mental health care services (Wijngaarden et al., 2003). Differences in caregiver burden could be caused by cultural characteristics. Cultures may differ in their appraisal of mental illness, with such appraisals ranging in attitude from acceptance and integration into society to stigmatization. Religious beliefs, beliefs regarding the origin of mental illness, and society's appraisal of the caregiver's role also play a part (Wijngaarden et al., 2003).

As the vast majority of previous studies have been conducted in Western cultures, it has been difficult to apply their findings to family caregivers in Asian countries. In a sample of caregivers of family members with schizophrenia in Japan and England, Nomura et al. reported that expressed emotion (EE) did not correlate significantly with caregiver burden. Decreased tendencies in caregivers' positive and negative emotional reactions towards family members, particularly in reactions to critical comments in the Japanese sample, were observed (Nomura et al., 2005).

2.2 Caregiver burden and cultural comparison

East Asian cultures based primarily on Confucian ideas have traditionally emphasized the importance of providing care for dependents. Studies of Chinese families in Malaysia have demonstrated that the stigma of relatives' mental illness has a strong and pervasive impact on family caregivers. To protect their families from "losing face", family caregivers often avoid talking about their relative's mental illness with extended family or friends (Chang & Horrocks, 2006). In a recent study on caregiver burden in China, families who perceived a higher level of caregiver burden were found to have poorer functioning, a lower health status, and lower satisfaction with social support. Social support was identified as the best predictor of caregiver burden (Chien et al., 2007). These results are similar to results obtained from our first survey of Japanese families (Hanzawa et al., 2008).

A cross-cultural and cross-national comparison of caregiver burden between Japan and Taiwan showed that Japanese respondents perceived a significantly stronger stigma for the parents and neighbors of a person with a mental illness presented in a vignette than did Taiwanese respondents (Shinfuku, 1998; Kurumatani et al., 2004). Haraguchi et al. reported that knowledge of mental illness and medication were greater in Japan than in China, but social distance for persons with mental illness was greater in Japan than in China. The reasons for these results include the fact that there are many advanced mental health care inpatient facilities as well as a few regional rehabilitation services in Japan. Also, Japan formerly had a long-term hospitalization system and hospital detention policy. In this policy, people with mental illnesses could be admitted involuntarily to a psychiatric hospital in order to receive treatment, without having exhibited violent behavior or suicide attempts (Haraguchi et al., 2009).

Korea is Japan's closest neighbor. A recent study of Korean relatives of patients with schizophrenia indicated that relatives with less knowledge about schizophrenia exhibited more inappropriate coping strategies and higher burdens (Lim & Ahn, 2003). Differences might exist in family caregivers' beliefs and attitudes among East Asian countries because the countries have varying socio-cultural and political backgrounds of mental health care systems.

2.2.1 Caregiver burden and the institutionalization rate for schizophrenia

In Japan, where the institutionalization rate for schizophrenia patients is the highest in the world, the number of psychiatric beds has not decreased during the last twenty years. Meanwhile, in Korea, a steady increase in the number of psychiatric beds has been observed over the past ten years (WHO, 2005). However, in Northeast Asian countries, little is known about the correlation between caregiver burden and socio-cultural and political factors. These factors may differ from country to country in the appraisal of the caregiver's role and coping strategies. Therefore, it is important to compare Japan and Korea to identify differences in socio-cultural and political backgrounds that could contribute to differences in caregiver burdens in these two countries. First, the tendency for Japanese families to exhibit decreased emotional expression towards family members as compared to Korean families was explored. Second, differences in religious beliefs and beliefs about the origin of mental illness and in the appraisal of the caregiver's role were identified through a cross-cultural comparison of Japan and Korea, with an emphasis on their histories of hospitalization and cultural differences.

2.2.2 A comparison of caregiver burden in Japan and Korea

In our first comparative study of Japanese and Korean family caregivers (Hanzawa et al., 2010a), members of the Federation of Families of People with Mental Illness in Japan and Korea were recruited and evaluated. Several differences between patients with schizophrenia of the two countries were observed. For example, although there were not significant differences of age and gender between Japanese and Korean sample, the percentage of patients who were frequently hospitalized (at least three times) were 34.3% and 59.8%, respectively. Clearly, Korean patients with schizophrenia were hospitalized more frequently over short periods of time. Differences in social activities over the past years and in the levels of living skills and care needs were also observed. Korean patients, compared to Japanese patients, had more opportunities to go out during the day and exhibited less impairment in the activities of daily living. However, Korean patients were hospitalized more frequently, and their families more strongly encouraged social participation. In a previous study, a multiple regression analysis identified the number of hospitalizations in the previous three years and kinship (mother/father/other) as significant predictors of caregiver burden (Caqueo & Gutierrez, 2006). The results of our second caregiver study did not identify the total number of hospitalizations in the previous year as a significant predictor in either country. However, the patients' social functioning and their care needs were both identified as significant predictors of caregiver burden in both Japan and Korea.

The results of our second caregiver study also suggest that, when compared to Korean families, constraints on the choice of caregiver in Japanese families (e.g., "I want care to be provided only by family members as much as possible") were significantly greater. In both countries, family caregiver burden was significantly correlated with an awareness of the fact that "the individual seems to feel uncomfortable with being cared for by someone outside the family". Thus, patients with schizophrenia in both countries are likely to avoid contact with non-family members and to isolate themselves from society. These factors were correlated with a greater caregiver role and an increased family caregiver burden.

In a study comparing five European countries, regional differences were identified in caregiver burden and support inside and outside the family (Magliano et al., 1998). Our results demonstrate slight differences in independent factors for caregiver burden between Japan and Korea. In Japan, families were more likely to have a greater caregiver burden if they agreed that "The individual seems to feel uncomfortable with being cared for by someone outside the family".

In Korea, family members are more likely to reluctantly allow someone outside the family to care for patients, so their family caregiver burden is lower. In the present study, about 70% of Korean families did not have someone who could provide care, which was a higher proportion than was observed in Japan. The results from Korea suggest that, when other family members also think that a patient with schizophrenia should be cared for by family, family members are more likely to collaborate in order to reduce caregiver burden. It might be difficult for family members to find caregivers who can provide care on behalf of the family, despite the fact that both Confucian ideas and the tradition of providing care to family members contribute to the reduction of caregiver burden.

Despite high family caregiver burden in both Japan and Korea, the present results demonstrate that patients and family members have a strong desire to restrict care to family members. The issue should be discussed further to reduce family caregiver burden, especially in relation to the quality of community mental health care services. For example, general practitioners, home-visit nurses, home help service providers, mutual support group members, other outreach services, and integrated assertive community services should provide advice for families having difficulties finding treatment and should suggest coping strategies for patients, especially during critical periods of relapse.

2.3 Public endorsement of stigma perception

Public endorsement of stigma affects many people. The following four groups are of special importance: people with mental illness, their families, service providers, and the general public. The harm that public stigma causes people who are labeled as mentally ill, as well as the harm to their family members and friends, is perhaps the greatest concern (Phelan et al., 1998; Link et al., 1999). Published research studies on public stigma (Magliano, 2004a), family stigma (Magliano et al., 2004b; Grausgruber et al., 2007), self-stigma (patient stigma) (Watson et al., 2007), and medical staff stigma (Lauber et al., 2005; Nordt et al., 2006) have elucidated the effects of stigma.

Italy is the country that has the longest experience with community-based psychiatric treatment. In the 20-year period following the promulgation of the 1978 Psychiatric Reform Law, a study revealed fearful attitudes in most of the general population in Italy toward mentally ill people. Twenty years later, a study of the coping strategies of "resignation" and "maintaining social interests" of families with schizophrenia showed a higher burden of care (Magliano et al., 1998). Now, approximately 30 years later, respondents who believe that patients with schizophrenia are unpredictable are more likely to report factors such as the use of alcohol and drugs as being involved in the development of the disorder (Magliano et al., 2004a). The concept of unpredictability is likely connected to the fear of violent behavior of patients with schizophrenia. The family's attitudes toward patients with schizophrenia may have a significant impact on patients' social adjustment and achievement of effective goals (Magliano et al., 2004b).

In Japan, the number of psychiatric beds has not decreased in the 20 years since community mental facilities were implemented across the country; thus, it is likely that attitudes regarding schizophrenia and its treatment have not changed. The public fear of assault from mentally ill patients has been expressed through community opposition to the opening of psychiatric institutions and through the general belief that these patients should be admitted to asylums. Japan is one of the few countries with almost no experience with psychiatric outreach treatment in the community for relatives of patients with delusional behavior that may occur during critical periods of schizophrenia. Previous research has demonstrated that Japanese respondents perceived a significantly stronger stigma for the parents and neighbors of a vignette case than did Taiwanese respondents (Shinfuku, 1998). It has been reported that the strong stigma among Japanese respondents may be a consequence of the limited experience of the general public with psychiatric patients in the community. This limited experience could be attributed to Japan's institutionalization rate for schizophrenia patients, which is the highest in the world (Kurumatani et al., 2004).

Few studies have investigated the relationship between caregiver experience and stigma in families with schizophrenia patients. For example, three out of every four Mexican-American schizophrenia patients live with their families, and a study of patient symptoms and attributes has shown a correlation between family care burden and stigma perception (Magaña et al., 2007). However, the effects of social stigma perception on the experience of families of patients with schizophrenia can vary between countries. Socio-cultural environmental factors regarding mentally ill persons can differ from country to country.

The relationship between burden and stigma in families of patients with schizophrenia remains unclear. No research had compared Japan and Korea with regard to the burden of care, stigma or social distance in families of patients with schizophrenia. In our second comparative study of Japanese and Korean family caregivers, stigma and care burden in families of patients with schizophrenia were compared in both countries (Hanzawa et al., 2009).

2.3.1 Caregiver experiences and stigma perception in Japan

When compared to Korea, the relationship between stigma perception and care burden among Japanese families is slightly more complicated. For example, Japanese families, compared to Korean families, tend to be "embarrassed" by the behaviors of schizophrenia patients, and they report "not feeling comfortable around a relative with schizophrenia". In addition, Japanese families are more likely to resist allowing people other than family members to care for schizophrenia patients. They are more likely to think that schizophrenia patients "feel uncomfortable with others entering his/her house" and "feel uncomfortable with being cared for by someone outside the family". Japanese families appear to be sensitive to schizophrenia patients' tendencies of "rejecting interactions with others and not wanting to be cared for by others besides family members at home, which is their safe space". Japanese families are also resistant to allowing others to take care of schizophrenia patients. Hence, a close family tie between schizophrenia patients and their families is suggested. The ratio of families who have access to people outside the family who could provide care in Japan was greater than half overall. However, even if Japanese families could find someone to provide care, they are more likely to care for schizophrenia patients on their own because they prefer not to have nonfamily members providing care.

In contrast to Korean families, Japanese families tend to believe that other people think chronic schizophrenia patients are "unpredictable and dangerous" and that "it is best to avoid them". Japanese families feel that "if they had a problem with schizophrenia, they would not tell anyone" and that "if a person had a problem with schizophrenia, he or she would not tell anyone", thus suggesting that their attitude is "it is best to hide schizophrenia in family members from others".

To summarize our third caregiver burden and family stigma study, Japanese families of patients with schizophrenia, compared to Korean families, are likely to perceive a stronger stigma from others and are more likely to think that schizophrenia should be hidden from others. Because they are "worried about what relatives and neighbors might think", they are more likely to take care of schizophrenia patients on their own. These findings are in agreement with the cognitive and behavioral characteristics of decision making by Japanese people (i.e., "make decisions to maintain harmony with others") (Radford & Nakane, 1991). However, the results of the present study show that the differences between Japan and Korea in terms of family nursing awareness and stigma perception by others do not significantly correlate with care burden. Interestingly, Japanese families that agreed with the statement "Want to provide care from family members only, without using home help services" experienced lower degrees of care burden.

Families of patients with schizophrenia have a more pessimistic view concerning their perception of stigma from the general public compared to their perception of their personal stigma. In particular, they hold pessimistic views concerning the ideas that people with schizophrenia are "dangerous", "unpredictable", and best to avoid. The findings of the present study indicate that family stigma of schizophrenia patients differs between Japan and Korea, especially regarding perceived stigma.

2.3.2 Caregiver experiences and stigma perception in Korea

While no significant difference existed in the perception of patients being dangerous to others, a personal stigma parameter, the family care burden exhibited a significant positive correlation in Korea. Furthermore, when compared to Japanese families, Korean families are more likely to believe that schizophrenia patients are "unpredictable", another personal stigma parameter. Care burden is great for Korean families with great personal stigma (e.g., "People with a problem like John's are unpredictable and dangerous"). Interestingly, in Korea, the family care burden was great for families who thought that the person in the vignette was discriminated against by families and by others in the community who were not willing to have the person in the vignette as their neighbor. Further, in Korea only, a significant positive correlation was observed between caregiver burden and the survey statement "If I had a problem like John's, I would not tell anyone". This correlation corresponds to the respondents' beliefs about other people's attitudes towards the person described in the vignette.

These results suggest that it will be necessary to provide support for lessening the care burden for families with personal stigma in Korea. For example, chronic schizophrenia patients are thought to be "dangerous and unpredictable", and that there are individuals who are unwilling to live near schizophrenia patients. Additionally, it is necessary to introduce family counseling programs and to provide individual family support to families who are likely to perceive social stigma. Such families are likely to agree with the statement "If I had a problem of schizophrenia, I would not tell anyone" and to believe "people in the community would be prejudiced". At the same time, the results in Korea suggest that strategies for lessening stigma in the local community, such as those exemplified by the statement "It is best to hide and not tell anyone about family members with schizophrenia", may eventually aid in lessening family care burden.

2.3.3 Coping strategies and stigma perception in East Asian countries

With the current shift to community-centered mental health services, considerable research on the family burden of caring for patients with schizophrenia has been conducted in European countries (Magliano et al., 1998). It has been reported that family burden and coping strategies can be influenced by cultural factors, and it has been suggested that family interventions should also have a social focus, with the aim of increasing the family social network and reducing stigma (Magliano et al., 1998).

Among Northeast Asian countries, it has been reported that, in Taiwan, caregiver anxiety is the highest of the five dimensions of primary family burden, followed by dependency of the patient and feelings of shame and guilt. In addition, home and family are considered to provide a person with the strongest sense of belonging and with a place to return to throughout life in Taiwanese society. Therefore, psychiatric patients traditionally live with their families (Hou et al., 2008). Similarly, it has been reported that approximately 80% of psychiatric patients in Japan and Korea live with their families (Hanzawa et al., 2009).

Pervasive negative attitudes and discriminatory treatment towards people with mental illness have been well documented in Northeast Asian countries and in Chinese societies. The particular manifestations of the stigma associated with schizophrenia are shaped by cultural meanings based on Confucianism. These cultural meanings are reflected in severe culture-specific expressions of stigma in Chinese societies (Yang, 2007). Yang et al. recently reported that psychiatric stigma in China is particularly pervasive and damaging. Rates of highly expressed emotion ("EE" or family members' emotional attitudes) are generally lower in China than in Western countries (Yang et al., 2010).

In our caregiver burden study, "resignation" and "maintaining social interests" were identified as coping strategies for the burden of care among mothers of patients with schizophrenia who were given the caregiver role by other family members (Hanzawa et al., 2008). In Korea, recent research has indicated that, among relatives of patients with schizophrenia, those relatives with less knowledge have more inappropriate coping strategies and higher burden (Lim & Ahn, 2003). Both Japan and Korea are located in Northeast Asia and have cultures based on Confucian ideas. These ideas include the tradition of providing care for dependents. In addition, Japan formerly had a long-term hospitalization system and a hospital detention policy that involuntarily admitted people with mental diseases to psychiatric hospitals. Thus, many inpatient psychiatric facilities exist today. Few people with serious mental disorders live in the community, given the stronger tendency for institutionalism in Japan than in other Asian countries (Kurihara et al., 2000; Warner, 2005). Consequently, the general public has little chance of coming into contact with patients with schizophrenia in everyday life (Haraguchi et al., 2009). It has been reported that Japanese respondents perceived significantly stronger stigmatization of the parents and neighbors of a vignette case than did Taiwanese respondents (Kurumatani et al., 2004).

Our fourth caregiver burden study compared Japan and Korea in terms of personal stigma and strategies for coping with a family member with schizophrenia, based on socio-cultural factors that could affect the care experience of families in Northeast Asian countries (Hanzawa et al., 2010b). The results clarified the similarities and differences in the characteristics of personal stigma towards a person with schizophrenia described in a vignette and in the coping strategies among families who belong to family support groups in Japan and Korea.

Differences in the attributes of the patients and their families were observed between Japan and Korea in the present study. For example, differences included the total number of hospitalizations (a higher number of hospitalizations was observed in Korea), patients' social functioning and care needs (Japanese patients had poorer functioning and required more care), optimal social involvement (the highest level of social involvement was observed in Korea), and an alternative caregiver in the family (fewer among families in Korea). Therefore, although Korean patients have a higher level of social functioning and social involvement, they also experience more hospital admissions. The results regarding coping strategies also suggest that patient social involvement with family is better in Korean families and that there are more strategies for coping with "patients' social involvement" in Korea. In contrast, although the overall scores for personal stigma were worse for Korean families, the personal stigma score for "If I had a problem like John's, I would not tell anyone" was worse for Japanese families. Thus, Japanese families of patients with schizophrenia would be more likely to hide their own mental illness from others, compared to Korean families. This likelihood is correlated with their high degree of "resignation" as a family coping strategy. Conversely, Korean families would be more likely to hide their mental illness through "avoidance" of a family member with schizophrenia.

These findings are in agreement with the cognitive and behavioral characteristics observed in cross-cultural qualitative studies that have explored the mental health beliefs and help-seeking attitudes of Korean-American parents of children with schizophrenia (Donnely, 2005). In the traditional Korean culture, a marriage signifies the union of two families rather than two individuals. Therefore, families of patients with mental illness worry about the marriage prospects for their other children if one child has a mental disorder. Furthermore, it has been reported that Korean families with children with mental disorders even object to visits by researchers. They fear that neighbors might recognize the investigators, thus revealing their child's mental disorder (Donnely, 2005). Family shame could be explained by the Confucian concept of filial piety, which states that no person should bring dishonor to the family (Sung, 1992). Children with schizophrenia are incapable of following the principles of filial piety, thus risking shame and violating traditional Korean beliefs (Donnely, 2005).

The results of the present correlation analysis demonstrated many differences between Japan and Korea in terms of factors that affect personal stigma and coping strategies. In particular, it is interesting to note that "coercion" and "avoidance" as family coping strategies were correlated with many aspects of personal stigma in Korea, but these strategies were not correlated with personal stigma in Japan. In contrast, the idea that "it is best to avoid people with a problem like John's" was correlated with almost all factors of coping in Korea.

3. Conclusion

Although the foundation of Confucian ideas and the tradition of providing care to family members are central to both Japanese and Korean cultures, unexpected similarities and differences between the two cultures were observed.

In both countries, patients with schizophrenia are likely to avoid contact with nonfamily members and to isolate themselves from society. These factors are correlated with a greater caregiver role and a worsening of the family caregiver burden.

However, Japanese families of patients with schizophrenia are more likely to perceive a strong stigma from others, compared to Korean families. Thus, they are more likely to think that schizophrenia should be hidden from others. Japanese families tend to cope with the stigma associated with schizophrenia through "resignation", in contrast to Korean families, who tend to cope through ineffective communication (e.g., "limited communication", "avoidance", and "coercion"). Furthermore, Japanese families are resistant to allowing others to care for a schizophrenic family member. A close family tie between schizophrenia patients and their families is suggested.

These findings suggest that Japanese mental health strategies should focus on providing effective support for reducing caregiver burden and for eliminating reliance on inappropriate coping strategies (e.g., "resignation", unwillingness to accept support from outside the family) for family members with schizophrenia inpatients and outpatients. This support is especially important for outpatients and their caregivers, as continued support from the early clinical stage through the chronic stage should be emphasized.

This issue should be discussed further in the context of community mental health care workers such as general practitioners, home-visit nurses, home help service providers, mutual support group members, and other outreach workers. Integrated assertive community services should be provided. These services are especially necessary during periods of relapse in patients living with chronic psychiatric illnesses. In future research, we will endeavor to summarize therapeutic encounters between family caregivers and health professionals. We will also examine available consultation and outreach treatments, such as using a multi-professional team approach in community settings. The team approach is suggested for optimal support of both patients with schizophrenia and their caregivers in Japan and South Korea.

4. Acknowledgments

The authors deeply appreciate the cooperation of the members of the Federation of Families of People with Mental Illness in Korea and Japan without which the study would never have been completed. I greatly appreciate Jeong-Kyu Bae, Professor of Daegu University for his assistance with this study. My thanks are also due to Yoshibumi Nakane, Emeritus professor of Nagasaki University, Yasuyuki Ohta, Professor of Nishikyushu University, and who gave many helpful suggestions. This study was partially supported by a Grant-in-Aid for Scientific Research (KAKENHI) (B) (22406036) (2010-12) from the Japanese Ministry of Education, Culture, Sports, Science and Technology (MEXT).

5. References

Caqueo, A., & Gutierrez, J. (2006) Burden of care in families of patients with schizophrenia. *Qual Life Res.* Vol.15: 719–724.

Chang, K.H. & Horrocks, S. (2006) Lived experiences of family caregivers of mentally ill relatives. *J. Adv. Nurs,* Vol.53: 435-443.

Chien, W.T., Chan, W.C., & Morrissey, J. (2007) The perceived burden among Chinese family caregivers of people with schizophrenia. *Journal of Clinical Nursing,* Vol.16: 1151-1161.

Donnelly, L.P. (2005) Mental health beliefs and help seeking behavior of Korean American parents of adult children with schizophrenia. *The Journal of Multicultural Nursing & Health,* Vol.11: 23-34.

Grausgruber, A., Meise, U., & Katschnig, H. (2007) Patterns of social distance towards people suffering from schizophrenia in Austria: a comparison between the general public, relatives and mental health staff. *Acta Psychiatrica Scandinavia,* Vol.115: 310-319.

Hanzawa, S., Tanaka, G., & Goto, M. (2008) Factors related to the burden for mothers of patients with schizophrenia; The impact of professional and social support network and family functioning on the burden. *Japanese Bulletin of Social Psychiatry,* Vol.16: 263-274.

Hanzawa, S., Bae, J.K., & Tanaka, H. (2009) Family stigma and care burden of schizophrenia patients: Comparison between Japan and Korea. *Asia-Pacific Psychiatry,* Vol.1: 120-129.

Hanzawa, S., Bae, J.K., & Tanaka, H. (2010a) Caregiver burden and coping strategies for patients with schizophrenia: Comparison between Japan and Korea. *Psychiat. Clin. Neurosci,* Vol.64: 77-386.

Hanzawa, S., Bae, J.K., & Tanaka, H. (2010b) Personal stigma and coping strategies in families of patients with schizophrenia: Comparison between Japan and Korea. *Asia-Pacific Psychiatry,* Vol.2: 105-113.

Haraguchi, K., Maeda, M., & Mei, Y.X. (2009) Stigma associated with schizophrenia: Cultural comparison of social distance in Japan and China. *Psychiat. Clin. Neurosci,* Vol.63: 153-160.

Hou, S.Y., Ke, C.L., & Su, Y.C. (2008) Exploring the burden of the primary family caregivers of schizophrenia patients in Taiwan. *Psychiat. Clin. Neurosci,* Vol.62: 508-514.

Kurihara, T., Kato, M., & Sakamoto, S. (2000) Public attitudes towards the mentally ill: A cross-cultural study between Bali and Tokyo. *Psychiat. Clin. Neurosci,* Vol.54: 547-552.

Kurumatani, T., Ukawa K., & Kawaguchi Y. (2004) Teachers' knowledge, beliefs and attitudes concerning schizophrenia: A cross-cultural approach in Japan and Taiwan. *Soc. Psychiatry Psychiatr. Epidemiol,* Vol.39: 402-409.

Lauber, C., Nordt, C., & Rosseler, W. (2005) Recommendations of mental health professionals and general population on how to treat mental disorders. *Soc Psychiatry Psychiatr Epidemiol,* Vol.40: 835-843.

Law Related to Mental Health and Welfare of the Person with Mental Disorder. (2006) Law No.94 dated June 23 2006, Tokyo, Japan.

Lee, S.K. (2009) East Asian Attitudes toward Death- A Search for the Ways to Help East Asian Elderly Dying in Contemporary America. *Perm J,* Vol.13: 55-60.

Lim, Y.M., & Ahn, Y.H. (2003) Burden of family caregivers with schizophrenic patients in Korea. *Appl Nurs Res,* Vol.16: 110-117.

Link, B.G., Phelan, J.C., & Bresnahan, M. (1999) Public conceptions of mental illness: Labels, causes, dangerousness, and social distance. *Am J Public Health,* Vol.89: 1328-1333.

Magaña, S.M., Ramírez, G.J.I., & Hernández, M.G. (2007) Psychological distress among latino family caregivers of adults with schizophrenia: the roles of burden and stigma. *Psychiatr Serv,* Vol.58: 378-384.

Magliano, L., Fadden, G., & Madianos, M. (1998) Burden on the families of patients with schizophrenia: results of the BIOMED I study. *Soc. Psychiatry Psychiatr. Epidemiol,* Vol.33: 405-412.

Magliano, L., Malangone, C., & Guarneri, M. (2001) The condition of families of patients with schizophrenia in Italy: burden, social network and professional support. *Epidemiol. Psichiatr. Soc,* Vol.10: 96-106.

Magliano, L., Marasco, C., & Fiorillo, A. (2002) The impact of professional and social network support on the burden of families of patients with schizophrenia in Italy. *Acta Psychiatr. Scand,* Vol.106: 291-298.

Magliano, L., Rosa, C.D., & Fiorillo, A. (2004) Perception of patients' unpredictability and beliefs on the causes and consequences of schizophrenia: A community survey. *Soc. Psychiatry Psychiatric Epidemiol,* Vol.39: 401-416.

Magliano, L., Fiorillo, A., & Rosa, C.D. (2004) Beliefs about Schizophrenia in Italy: A Comparative Nationwide Survey of the General Public, Mental Health Professionals, and Patients' Relatives. *Can. J. Psychiatry,* Vol. 49: 322-330.

Mental Health Act in Taiwan, 2007.

Nomura, H., Inoue, S., & Kamimura, N. (2005) A cross-cultural study on expressed emotion in carers of people with dementia and schizophrenia: Japan and England. *Soc. Psychiatry Psychiatr. Epidemiol,* Vol.40: 564-570.

Nordt, C., Rosseler, W., & Lauber, C. (2006) Attitudes of Mental Health Professionals toward People with Schizophrenia and Major Depression. *Schizophrenia Bulletin,* Vol.32: 709-714.

Phelan J.C., Bromet E.J., & Link B.G. (1998) Psychiatric illness and family stigma. *Schizophr. Bull.* Vol.24: 115–126.

Radford, M.H.B. & Nakane, Y. (1991) Ishi-kettei-koui: Culture and Decision Making Behaviour, 1st ed. Human TY, ISBN4-938632-29-2, Tokyo (in Japanese)

Roick, C., Heider, D., & Toumi, M. (2006) The impact of caregivers' characteristics, patients' conditions and regional differences on family burden in schizophrenia: a longitudinal analysis. *Acta Psychiatr. Scand,* Vol.114: 363-374.

Roick, C., Heider, D., & Bebbington, P. (2007) Burden on caregivers of people with schizophrenia: comparison between Germany and Britain. *Br. J. Psychiatry,* Vol.190: 333-338.

Shinfuku, N. (1998) Mental health services in Asia: International perspective and challenge for the coming years. *Psychiatry and Clinical Neurosciences,* Vol.52: 269-274.

Sung, K.T. (1992) Motivations for parent care: the case of filial children in Korea. *Int J Aging Hum Dev.* Vol.34: 109-124.

Warner, R. (2005) Local project of the World Psychiatric Association Programme to Reduce Stigma and Discrimination. *Psychiatr. Serv,* Vol.56: 570-575.

Watson, A.C., Corrigan, P., & Larson, J.E. (2007) Self-Stigma in People with Mental Illness. *Schizophr Bull,* Vol.33: 1312-1318.

van Wijngaarden, B., Schene, A., & Koeter, M, (2003) People with Schizophrenia in Five Countries: Conceptual Similarities and Intercultural Differences in Family Caregiving. *Schizophr Bull,* Vol.29: 573-586.

World Health Organization. (2005) Mental Health Atlas-2005. World Health Organization, Geneva, Switzerland.

Yang, L.H. (2007) Application of mental illness stigma theory Chinese societies: synthesis and new directions. *Singapore Med J*, Vol.48, pp.977-985.

Yang, L.H., Phillips, M.R., & Lo, G. (2010) "Excessive Thinking" as Explanatory Model for Schizophrenia: Impacts on Stigma and "Moral" Status in Mainland China. *Schizophr. Bull*, Vol.36: 836-45.

Part 2

Clinical Research on Cognition in Schizophrenia

Schizophrenia and Social Cognition: From Conceptual Bases to Therapeutic Approaches

Luciana de Carvalho Monteiro, Paula Andreia Martins,
Marisa Crivelaro and Mario Rodrigues Louzã
Institute of Psychiatry, Clinicas Hospital,
University of São Paulo School of Medicine
Brazil

1. Introduction

Social cognition has developed independently from neurosciences, with a focus on understanding socioemotional phenomena, i.e., the relationship between the analysis of the social context, of cognitive processing and its base in the central nervous system. It evolved from studies with animals, including experiments such as competing for food, protection strategies and adaptative responses to the social environment of certain species, and application of the resulting knowledge to a better understanding of the evolution of social cognition in human beings. Such studies showed that the development of complex behavior was associated with the increase in the level of response imposed by the environment. This resulted in the ability to deal with unexpected situations and build representations of the relationship with oneself and with others, in order to govern social behavior. Thus, behaviors such as cooperation and selflessness became a key factor in group interaction (Adolphs, 2001, Emery & Clayton, 2009).

Flaws in social human functioning, including communication with others, preservation of employment, interactions in community and ability to live independently, can be observed in serious metal disorders, such as schizophrenia. Understanding the mechanisms involved in such flaws, differentiating them from basic cognitive deficits, is of the utmost importance both for establishing investigation strategies into dysfunctions in social cognition, and for the development of therapeutic intervention programs.

1.1 Concept of social cognition

Social cognition is the capacity to identify, manipulate and adapt behavior in accordance with socially relevant cues detected and processed in a certain context of the environment. To that end, it requires an underlying neural system that manages everything from the stimulus input (perception) to the final result of the process, i.e., manifestation of the adaptive social behavior.

Social cognition guides both automatic and intentional behavior, together with a wide range of other basic cognitive processes, modulating the behavioral response. However, although it is generally established that the basic cognitive processes, such as attention, memory and executive functions are necessary for social cognition, they are considered different constructs, as they utilize semi-independent processing systems (Penn et al, 1997; Adophs, 2001; Couture et al, 2006).

Neurocognition and social cognition differ in that the latter is a mediator between neurocognition and social functioning. The distinction between social cognition and neurocognition is the focus of studies not only of social psychologists, but also of researchers in evolution biology and primate behavior. These emphasize the fact that the mechanisms involved in processing information in the human mind are not designed to perform tasks arbitrarily, but rather, to solve specific biological issues imposed by the physical, ecological and social environment encountered by our ancestors in the course of the evolution of the species (Cosmides, 1989 as cited in Penn, 1997)

It may be concluded that neurocognition and social cognition are different manners to comprehend human behavior. Social cognition consists of a mental operation, which is at the core of social functioning, involving the capacity to perceive the intention and disposition of others in a certain context. This includes abilities in emotional and social perception, attribution of causality and empathy, and reflects the influence of the social context (Penn et al., 1997; Couture et al.; 2006).

1.2 Components of social cognition

Social cognition can be understood through a conceptual model which involves four specific domains: theory of mind (ToM), attribution style (AS), emotion recognition (ER) and social perception (SP), as indicated in Table 1.

Theory of Mind (ToM)	Ability to understand that others display states of mind that differ from mine and to make inferences based on the content of such mental states.
Attribution Style (AS)	Particular tendency to explain the causes of events in own life
Emotion Recognition (ER)	Ability to infer emotional information from emotional expressions, voice pitch and/or prosody.
Social Perception (SP)	Ability to extract manifest behavioral cues within a certain social context. It includes the ability to understand social rules and conventions.

Table 1. Components of Social Cognition.

1.2.1 Theory of Mind

The term "Theory of Mind" (ToM) was initially coined by primatologists Premack and Woodruff in a seminal paper published in 1978 which suggested that chimpanzees were able to infer the mental state of other individuals of the same species (Brüne & Brüne-Cohrs, 2006). Over time, the term was adopted by developmental psychology to describe the ontogenic evolution of the mental process in infancy and adolescence.

In psychopathology, the concept of dysfunction of the ToM has been increasingly used in studies involving autistic children. It has been observed that both autistic children and adults (including Asperger's Syndrome), present significant difficulties to apprehend the mental state of other individuals.

Currently, the study of the ToM in other mental disorders has caught the attention of researchers in areas such as schizophrenia and its relation with other aspects of cognition and symptoms, as well as its effect on social behavior (Brüne & Brüne-Cohrs, 2006; Brüne, 2005). This concept has been a focal point for cognitive psychology, which has dedicated itself to developing several models to explain the ToM. Among them, the Baron-Cohen model (1996) conceives the existence of four cerebral modules which interact to produce the "mind reading" system of human beings (Table 2).

1. Intentionality module	Capacity to interpret a stimulus as intentional based on a desire and goal formulation.
2. Gaze direction module	Ability to perceive another individual's gaze, and interpret whether this "gaze" is perceiving the same as the individual's own gaze.
3. Shared attention module	Ability to establish relations with own self, with other individuals and with the perceived objects, i.e. "do you and I perceive the same?".
4. Theory of Mind module	Ability to integrate the three modules above - perception, desire, intention - and the construction of coherent theoretical beliefs, which enable comprehension of the behavior of another individual and, thus, define and direct the individual's own behavior.

(Monteiro et al., 2010)

Table 2. Cerebral modules responsible for the ToM, proposed by Baron-Cohen (1996).

Developmental psychology devoted itself to comprehending the origin of this ability in children and how it organizes itself in the several stages of human development.

The ontogenesis of the ToM does not differ significantly from the maturity of other cerebral functions, also following a sequence of acquisitions (eg.: to sit, to stand and to walk) (Brüne & Brüne-Cohrs, 2006). Thus, at around twelve months old, the child is already able to perceive his/herself, to perceive the agent (eg. his/her mother) and to perceive the object (shared attention), which, according to the Baron-Cohen's conceptual model, includes a fundamental element for the existence of the ToM. After this period, the child progressively develops more complex abilities, such as distinguishing between the representation of a real event and of a hypothetical situation, the perception of his/her own reflex in the mirror and discrimination of false beliefs.

The concept of ToM includes a most fundamental dimension of human awareness for social behavior. It is via this cognitive resource that humans can achieve more sophistication in the relations and communication among individuals of their own group, as well as individuals from other groups, enabling recognition and interpretation of expressions such as irony, concealment, suffering, interest and deceit. Based on such information, the individual is able to anticipate the ideas the other is forming of him/herself, predict events and make critical decisions in the social environment (Monteiro et al., 2010).

1.2.2 Attribution style

Attribution Style is the explanation found by an individual for the positive and/or negative consequences of events in his/her own life.

Most people attribute positive outcomes to themselves (internal attribution) and negative outcomes such as guilt, flaws or other threats, to external factors (external attribution). The subject processes a stimulus, attributes a style to it and reaches a certain causality conclusion.

A study model of Attribution Style stemming from research in social psychology and experimental clinic was the attribution style in depression, which is related to prolonged exposure to uncontrollable aversive events, which result in motivational, cognitive and behavioral deficits (Schill & Marcus, 1998). In this form of attribution style, individuals believe that there is no way positive outcomes can be achieved or aversive consequences prevented (Seligman, 1990).

The classic pessimistic attribution style can be observed in individuals who tend to explain negative outcomes or failures as internal attribution processes, i.e., blaming themselves, as opposed to external attribution styles in which failure is attributed to the environment. As a rule, the interpretation of these internal causes tends to be stable (continuous) and generalized. Conversely, an individual with an optimistic attribution style interprets negative outcomes, i.e., failure, to external, unstable and specific factors (Peterson & Seligman, 1984). The style that can be observed in depression seems not to be state-dependent, as it tends to remain even upon remission of symptoms. This tendency can be deemed as a trace of susceptibility to depression (Just et al., 2001).

Based on studies involving depressed patients, one can assume that an attribution style can help understand the behaviors and consequences which affect the performance and actions of individuals within the social context.

1.2.3 Emotion recognition

Emotion recognition is the ability to infer information from emotional expressions identified in the human face, voice inflection and/or prosody, which is the emotional pitch of human speech.

While there are differences in social rules and customs dictated by culture, facial expressions are universally recognized. Happiness, sadness, anger, fear, repulse, surprise and possibly contemplation are universally detectable emotions. However, unlike universal emotions, social emotions such as guilt, shame and arrogance are specific for each culture (Kohler et. al., 2004a, b).

Emotion plays an important role in preparing action; for that, it is necessary to organize coherent behavioral strategies which rely on efficient collection of information from the environment.

Perception of faces and emotional expressions involve distinct cerebral structures and neurobiological circuits, and are therefore perceived as two separate processes which interact with each other, and are characterized as physiological and cognitive.

The physiological process seems to be associated with the amygdala, due to its influence in the emotional content of complex perception stimuli, although it is not the only structure involved. The basal nucleus, the one with the largest interconnection with the ventromedial prefrontal cortex, acts in pairing social cues with the appropriate social context, preparing the body for the appropriate behavior and actions (Emery & Amaral 2000).

The cognitive process consists of conscious experience, pairing stimulus and the corresponding corporal response. This system is regulated by superior brain areas, the cortex of the cyngulus and the frontal lobes.

One of the manners by which an individual can produce, recognize and interpret emotional expressions in the face is by reproducing such expressions in his own body and detecting the feeling it triggers (Adolphs, 1999). This ability is an important component in interpersonal communication, the expressions being used to convey an emotional state, so that the apt "reading of emotions" can supply impressions to lead the individual to act within an appropriate social context (Fuentes et al., 2010).

1.2.4 Social perception

Social perception is the ability to pick up cues from behaviors within a given social context and includes the ability to understand social rules and conventions. It consists of forming impressions of others, through the perception of cultural codes and rules that regulate the appropriate actions and behaviors within a given social context. The ability to identify the typical behaviors of each context and culture reduces the occurrence of gridlocks in the relationship among individuals in a given group (Del Prette & Del Prette, 2009, Rocca et al., 2010).

Social perception enables the appropriate interpretation of the social world and the control over it. It plays an important role in decision-making and in situations requiring interaction with other individuals. It is with basis on this "social reading" that the formation of mental schemes is structured.

1.3 Neuroanatomical substrates and information processing

The neural substrates involved in the processing of social stimuli include the cortical regions of the temporal lobe, while the amygdala, the right somatosensory cortex, the orbitofrontal cortex and the cyngulate are involved in connecting the perception of the social stimulus to motivation, emotion and cognition (Adolphs, 2001; Ochsner, 2004).

The medial prefrontal cortex is a crucial component in mediating neural systems of perception of the social context, promoting adaptation of behavior (Krueger and cols. 2009).

Social reasoning and decision-making are associated with the ventromedial prefrontal cortex, while emotional awareness of facial expression involves the amygdala. The ability to simulate and empathize is associated with the right somatosensorial cortex, while automatic response is related to the insula (Bechara, Damasio & Damasio, 2003).

Social Cognition, together with a wide range of other basic cognitive processes, such as attention, memory, language and the executive functions, govern automatic and intentional behavior, regulating the behavioral response (Penn et al., 1997; Couture et. al., 2006).

Social information processing is proposed by Sapute and Lieberman (2006), from a neural base model divided into *reflexive systems* and *reflective systems* (Table 3). The reflexive system operates through automatic processes, whereas the reflective system operates through controlled processes.

Reflexive System (automatic processes)	Reflective System (controlled processes)
Parallel Processing	Serial Processing
Fast Operations	Slow Operations
Slow Learning	Fast Learning
Non Reflective Awareness	Reflective Awareness
More ancient Filogenetic Structure	Newer Filogenetic Structure
Representation of symetrical relations	Representation of asymetrical relations
Representation of ordinary cases	Representation of special cases and abstract concepts

Table 3. Characteristics of the Reflexive and Reflective Systems (Monteiro and Louzã 2010).

The automatic processes involve the amygdala, the basal ganglia, the ventromedial prefrontal cortex, the dorsal anterior cingulate cortex and the temporal lateral cortex, being these regions involved in encoding traits and evaluating the implications of an observed behavior (Monteiro e Louzã, 2010).

The prefrontal lateral, the posterial parietal, the prefrontal medial cortices, the anterior rostral cingulate and the areas of the medial temporal lobe, including the hippocampus, are involved in voluntary processes, referred to as the reflexive system. These regions are responsible for exploring the inferred objects in the mind, and also for apprehending the situational information added to previous knowledge, in order to alter the interference of observed behaviors.

Automatic processing does not require much effort, for which reason it is considered qualitatively different from controlled processing. In automatic processing, the evaluation is out of the realm of conscience, does not receive attention modulation and is hard to regulate and control. The processing occurs in a parallel manner, involving tasks already known and performed, and thus considered stereotyped and automatic.

Controlled processing is intentional, voluntary or requires effort. It occurs in consciousness and is deemed slow; regulation is accessible and requires attention resources. The processing is done in series, so that information is processed in a step by step manner, enabling the individual to deal with new and difficult tasks, never before performed. Processing appears later in development terms, and involves declaratory language, reasoning and the ability to reflect and ponder. It utilizes complex levels of cognitive processing, such as: semantics, synthesis and abstraction.

1.4 Evaluation paradigm

The conceptual model of social cognition has been used to investigate both social competence functioning, through standardized instruments, and the structures involved in this functioning, through neuroimaging studies.

The most cited instruments in the current literature according to each cognitive domain are listed in Table 4.

Social Cognition Domains	Tests
Emotion Recognition	Bell-Lysaker Emotion Recognition Test, Facial Affect recognition, Facial Emotion Identification Test , Facial Expression of Emotion, Penn Emotion Acuity Test, Pictures of Facial Affect, Videotape Affect Perception Test, Emotional Differentiation Task, Facial Emotion Discrimination Test, Voice Emotion Discrimination Test , Mayer-Salovey-Caruso Emotional Intelligence Test, Prosody Task , Vocal Affect Recognition and Voice Emotion Identification
Social Perception	Half-Profile of Nonverbal Sensitivity (PONS), Social Behavior Sequencing Task (SBST), Social Perception Scale (SPS), Picture Arrangement Subtest (WAIS), Situational Feature Recognition Test, Schema Component Sequencing Task, Social Cue Recognition Task, Social Cue Recognition Task-revised, Social Stimuli Sequencing Task and Comprehension Subtest (WAIS)
Theory of Mind (ToM)	Attribution of Intention errors, Advanced ToM Scale, Hinting Task, The Awareness of Social Inference Test (TASIT), ToM stories, Tom Picture Stories, Tom Vignettes, Faux Pas Task, Eyes Test and Implicit Mentalizing Task
Attributional Style	Ambiguous Intentions Hostility Questionnaire (AIHQ)
Social Functioning	Nurses' Observation Scale for Inpatient Evaluation (NOSIE), Personal and Social Performance Scale (PSP), Social Adjustment Scale (SAS), Social Behavioral Scale (SBS), World Health Organization Disability Assessment Schedule (WHODAS)

(M. M. Kurtz & C. L. Richardson, 2011; A-K.J. Fett et al., 2011)

Table 4. Selected Tests for the Social Cognition Assessment.

2. Social cognition and schizophrenia

Over recent years there has been a growing interest in the study of Social Cognition impairments in schizophrenia. These studies have explored the social cognition of individuals at ultra-high risk to develop psychosis (especially schizophrenia), the first psychotic episode and chronic schizophrenia. Besides, some studies have also measured social cognition impairments in persons with high risk to schizophrenia (relatives of patients, especially first degree relatives, including parents and children of schizophrenic patients) and individuals with schizotypy.

The term ultra-high risk (UHR) has been used to define individuals that fulfill operational criteria for "psychosis risk syndrome", measured with the use of structured interviews such as the The Structured Interview for Prodromal Symptoms and the Scale of Prodromal Symptoms - SIPS/SOPS (Miller, 2003) or the Comprehensive Assessment of At Risk Mental State - CAARMS (Addington, 2004). Sometimes, the expression "prodromal state" or "prodrome" or "prodromal phase" is also used to refer to UHR individuals.

Current findings have demonstrated that individuals at prodromal state, ultra high risk and first psychotic episode may already present impairments, which can still be found in the remission period and/or symptoms relapse.

2.1 Studies in prodromal, first-episode and chronic schizophrenia

2.1.1 Attribution style

Psychotic patients have a tendency to attribute negative events to an external agent, and this externalization trend is associated with delusions. The tendency to externalize is particularly evident in persecutory and self-reference delusions, in which individuals interpret the intentions of others as personal and negative (Janssen et. al., 2006). Aakre (2009) studied the attribution style of currently paranoid patients, comparing them to paranoid patients in remission, non-paranoid patients in remission and healthy controls, and observed that currently paranoid patients demonstrated a greater tendency to "external-personal attributions" to negative events. The other groups of patients also presented a greater tendency to adopt internal-personal and internal-universal attributions to negative events. Mizhara (2008) evaluated patients with schizophrenia, with schizoaffective disorder and with schizophreniform disorder, and verified a direct relation between the intensity of the psychopathology and an internalizing attribution style.

Krstev (1999) studied 62 first-episode patients and observed a lower rate of suspiciousness (measured through BPRS) and more depression (Beck Depression Inventory) predicted higher scores of internal attributions for negative events. An et al. (2010) observed an association between persecutory symptoms and perceived hostility bias in first-episode patients.

The attribution style bias associated with paranoid symptoms may not only be present in first-episode patients, but also before the beginning of frank psychotic events, and evolves upon diagnozing the individual. Patients with schizophrenia perceive hostility more acutely, associated with positive symptoms; UHR individuals present less bias to perceive hostility and react aggressively to ambiguous situations. This low tendency to aggressiveness, however, could be a distinct trait of UHR patients. These also presented a tendency to avoid hostile situations refraining from approaching another person, and have a tendency to blame such person. (An et. al., 2010). However, Janssen (2006) did not observe alterations of attribution style in first-degree relatives of non-affective psychosis patients and in individuals with sub-clinical psychotic experiences.

2.1.2 Theory of Mind (ToM)

Studies have demonstrated that schizophrenic patients present significant impairments in the ability to infer the mental state of other individuals. These deficits are more significant in the acute phase of the disease, and seem to persist during remission periods. The alterations observed may indicate a possible marker of schizophrenia (Sprong, 2009; Bora, 2009).

Chung et.al. (2007) suggest that mild deficits in social cognition in the prodomic phase of schizophrenia are verified, and could be attributed to a prefrontal dysfunction. Some studies have demonstrated cognitive impairment in ToM tasks in ultra high risk individuals, and these deficits could be risk markers evolving over time, to differentiate functional and clinical deterioration (Bonshtein, 2006).

There is a significant association between ultra high risk and impairments in ToM tasks, verified through errors committed by such individuals in false belief tasks of first and second degree, although these individuals present equivalent performance in superior order tasks, which are not significantly different from the performance of individuals with schizophrenia and the good performance of healthy adult controls. Evidence of impairment of brain circuits associated with mentalization were evaluated by means of functional magnetic resonance, comparing the intensity of activation of different areas of the brain during the performance of ToM tasks by the families of schizophrenic individuals, with and without a history of psychotic symptoms, and controls. The first ultra high risk group activated several areas of the prefrontal cortex less intensely when compared to the second group, which could suggest, albeit inconclusively, that ToM deficits are trace-dependent (Tonetti et. al., 2008).

Koelkebeck, (2010), investigated ToM in first-episode schizophrenia patients and healthy controls, and analyzed the relationship with neuropsychological and psychopathological functioning. Alhtough first-episode patients did not present differences when compared with the control group in response to videos with random movement, moderate cognitive deficits were observed in inaccurate description used and less ToM-related vocabulary when responding to socially complex ToM video sequences. Deficits in ToM are present from the initial stage of the disease, and the impairments verified may be independent from the clinical history, from alexithymia and from empathy.

Bertrand (2007) assessed ToM in first-episode of schizophrenia spectrum psychosis and healthy controls. Differences were observed between the groups in the Hinting Task and the Four Factor Test of Social Intelligence, but the Four Factor Test of Social Intelligence demonstrated the strongest effect in the group, and the effects observed remain significant. The findings did not present correlation with the intensity of symptoms.

Review and meta-analysis show that ToM deficits are more intense in the acute phase of the disease, although it persists even during periods of remission. Healthy relatives of individuals with schizophrenia and individuals with high scores of schizotypy also present deficits of ToM. Intellectual deficits seem to influence the impairment of ToM in patients in remission (Bora 2009, Bora et al. 2009).

Achim et al. (2010) evaluated the relationship between levels of empathy, performance in mentalization and clinical symptoms of first psychotic episode, and healthy individuals. These results were also compared with previous studies in patients with chronic schizophrenia through meta-analysis. The authors observed that the evaluations of the interpersonal reaction index (IRI) did not differ significantly between first-episode patients and the control group. In first-episode patients, there was no correlation between IRI and positive and negative symptoms, or symptoms of general psychopathology, but a significant negative correlation between the Liebowitz Social Anxiety Scale and Perspective taking was observed. A positive correlation between the Empathic concern subscale and our ToM task was also observed. Patients in first-episode of psychosis presented lower impairment of empathy than chronic schizophrenic patients.

The literature review carried out by Tonelli et al (2009) identified fifteen studies which evaluated schizotypal traces and the relations between vulnerability to psychosis and alterations in ToM processing. Most studies suggest that individuals with high scores in schizotypy scales, relatives of schizophrenic patients, who present deficits in ToM processing, could suggest a dependent character trait. Some studies have confirmed the hypothesis that schizophrenic individuals with a predominance of negative symptoms and disorganization, score lower in ToM tasks than individuals with a predominance of positive symptoms. ToM alterations in schizophrenic patients could derive from primary general cognitive deficits, since the brain structures involved in processing Social Cognition and ToM are also called upon for processing other non social cognitive functions (Tonelli et al. 2009).

2.1.3 Emotion recognition

Difficulties in emotion recognition are present before the manifestation of psychosis in high risk individuals (Thompson et al 2011). Edwards (2001) evaluated facial and prosody emotion recognition in individuals with first episode psychosis and controls. It was observed that the participants did not differ in the understanding of the words used to describe emotions. However, slight but consistent deficits in the recognition of fear and sadness in both channels of communication were observed. These findings can suggest a characteristic deficit, consistent with dysfunction of the amygdala in schizophrenia and related psychosis (Amminger 2011). These data suggest that deficits in facial emotion recognition may serve as an endophenotype for schizophrenia (Addington et. al., 2008, Li et. al., 2010).

The study of Kohler et al. (2009) revealed that schizophrenic patients present deficits in emotion recognition, irrespective of the type of task and factors that may act as moderators of the impairment observed, such as the clinical symptoms and anti-psychotic treatment. Patients with schizophrenia present flaws in the recognition of fear and in the interpretation of social cues in faces. Recent studies have demonstrated limbic hyperactivity in these patients when they see nonfearful and fearful faces, as compared with basal values. Hyperactivity of the amygdala can also be detected when individuals with schizophrenia cannot adequately recognize fearful faces (Morris et al., 2009).

Eack et al. (2010) suggest that deficits in emotion recognition in schizophrenic and ultra high risk individuals could be related to difficulties in visual perception, which is also observed in individuals with schizophrenia. In this respect, alterations in neurocognition can interfere with the ability to discriminate emotions, consequently impairing social cognition. Sachs et al. (2004) compared patients with schizophrenia and healthy volunteers in computerized tasks of recognition of emotion. They were also tested with a standard neuropsychological battery and rated for positive and negative symptoms. Patients with schizophrenia performed more poorly than controls in all the tasks of emotion recognition. The most significant difficulties were verified in discriminating happiness, differentiating sad from happy faces, and facial memory. The latter may be correlated with the severity of the negative symptoms. These findings suggest that the notion of difficulty in emotion recognition in schizophrenia may be associated with specific cognitive deficits.

Addington (2006) evaluated patients with first episode psychosis, schizophrenia patients with multiple episodes of psychosis and controls. The individuals were evaluated in two tasks of facial recognition, a complete cognitive battery and a measure of social functioning. Both patients were clearly impaired when compared with the controls in social cognition and recognition of facial emotions. Significant associations between the functioning of facial recognition and recognition of facial emotions were observed in all three groups. However, there was no evidence that the recognition of facial emotions partially affects the mediation between the relations of social and cognitive functioning.

Two recent reviews highlight some points in the deficit of emotion recognition in schizophrenia. There is controversy as regards the kind of emotion whose deficit is more aggravated, while in others, any kind of emotion is poorly identified. The association with clinical symptoms is likewise unclear, and both positive and negative symptoms could influence emotion recognition. The fact that the deficit of emotion recognition is pervasive in the disease from the beginning and remains along its course suggests that it is a trait-marker of schizophrenia (Morris et al. 2009, Marwick e Hall 2008).

2.1.4 Social perception

There are few studies in this area, although researchers have shown interest in exploring the perception of social interactions in individuals with psychoses. Studies have demonstrated impairments in schizophrenia, usually expressed in a more subtle manner in first-episode and ultra high risk individuals. Couture (2008) evaluated UHR individuals, schizophrenic patients and controls, proposing a task in which the participants made social judgments of unknown faces. The findings demonstrated that the ultra high risk group classifies unreliable faces as more reliable. However, they did not present differences when compared to the control group when judging reliable faces. Ultra high risk individuals classified dishonest faces as positive, more frequently that the controls. Ultra high risk individuals presented partial response to unreliable faces, when compared with schizophrenic individuals and controls (Thompson et. al., 2011).

Green (2011) evaluated the relationship between the domains of social cognition: social perception and emotion recognition and neurocognition in high risk, first-episode, and schizophrenic individuals and controls. The authors observed impairment in cognitive performance and in all the areas of social cognition in all the groups of the sample. Performance differences between the groups were comparable between the phases of the disease, not evidencing progress or improvement. Pinkham (2007) evaluated social perception and emotion recognition in ultra high risk individuals, individuals in the early stages of the schizophrenia spectrum, chronic schizophrenic patients and healthy controls. Ultra high risk individuals did not differ significantly from the control group. However, individuals in the early stages of the disease and chronic schizophrenics presented significant deficits, demonstrating poorer performance than controls, but not differing from each other, although there is evidence that deficits in social skills can be observed from the onset of the disease. The findings suggest that deficits in social perception skills can be a vulnerability marker for schizophrenia.

Although the results point out deficits in ultra high risk and schizophrenic individuals, one must understand the variations in the course of the disease, as well as observe factors such as: stress, previous experiences with the disorder and current experiences, which may be dependent on or independent from the progress of the disorder. Longitudinal studies in this area are required to better explain the course and severity of these difficulties (Couture et al., 2008).

2.2 The impact of social cognition impairments on functioning

Social cognition is a specialized area of cognition, which enables the individual to adapt to group or social life. Impairments in social cognition result in difficulties in the social functioning of individuals with schizophrenia.

Alterations in social cognition result in flaws in these individuals' social functioning, obstructing their independent living, impacting decision-making and situations in which the interaction with other individuals is required. These flaws result in day to day difficulties, such as preservation of employment and community life, due to the inability to interpret and have control over the social world around them. It is based on this "social reading" that the mental schemes are structured. For these individuals, there is impairment in relationships, in interpreting a given stimulus, in perceiving another individual's gaze, in the formation of relationships with themselves and with others, in integrating perception, desire, beliefs and intentions.

The individual who presents defective processing of ToM is prevented from subjectively representing an important variable of reality, the mental state of others, impairing the distinction between subjectivity and objectivity. Deprived of the ability to accurately interpret the mental content of others, attributes to them feelings and thoughts that may be offensive, threatening or seductive, thus representing a possible mechanism that favors the appearance of paranoid and erotomaniac delusions.

Deficits in attribution style lead these individuals to perceiving hostility more intensely. Ambiguous situations in which the contextual cues are scarce may lead an individual to interpret the environment or people as socially threatening, provoking avoidance behaviors and ensuing isolation, since he/she believes that others do not have good intentions, an additional fuel for paranoid ideation (Bentall et al., 2001).

The ability for social play is dependent upon the systematization and hierarchization of a series of cues supplied in each social context. This is subject to how the individual has access to the mental universe of others with all the network of contextualization it requires. Emotion plays an important role in preparation for action, which requires organizing coherent behavioral strategies, and which, in turn, depend on the efficient perception of environmental cues.

Different cultures exist and diverge in terms of social rules and customs. But when it comes to facial expressions, emotion is universally recognized. A deficit in this kind of cognition, prevents the individual from inferring emotional information from perceived emotional expressions, voice pitch and/or prosody, consequently preventing him/her from reproducing the facial expression in his/her own body, and detecting the feeling it triggers. This results in difficulties to identify the directions to be followed within an adequate social context (Fuentes, et. al., 2010).

Deficient functioning of social perception impairs the perception of social cues expressed in the behavior within a given social environment. Thus, the individual is unable to understand social rules and conventions which govern behavior within specific social contexts.

3. Therapeutic approaches

Therapeutic interventions that improve deficits in social cognition are of the utmost importance, considering the impact that these flaws have in functioning, quality of life and socio-economic cost of the disease, be it in its initial stages or in the chronic state.

3.1 Intervention models

Three treatment strategies have been used: a) psychotherapeutic rehabilitation aimed at reducing the psychotic symptoms and functional improvement;) specific medication targeted at the cognitive mechanisms related to the psychotherapeutic rehabilitation; and c) use of anti-psychotic medication to reduce symptoms and facilitate the patient's engagement in the cognitive rehabilitation (Swerdlow, 2011).

3.2 Pharmacological interventions

There is some evidence in different meta-analyses, that antipsychotic drugs improve neurocognition in schizophrenic patients. First generation antipsychotics improved neurocognition with a mean effect size of 0.22, with a range between 0.13-0.29 for the majority of cognitive functions (Mishara and Goldberg, 2004). Other authors concluded that second generation antipsychotics are superior to first generation antipsychotics, improving overall cognitive function with an effect size of 0.24. They also concluded that different antipsychotics might have differential effects on the different cognitive domains (Woodward et al. 2005). Thornton et al. (2006) examined the influence of different antipsychotics on long-term memory of schizophrenic, schizoaffective and schizophreniform patients and showed that antipsychotics with less anticholinergic effect produce a more robust improvement of the long-term memory. Other agents (e.g., cholinergic, glutamatergic, dopaminergic) showed conflicting results so that there is no clear evidence that these drugs improve cognition in schizophrenia (Barch 2010).

There are relatively few studies that addressed the influence of antipsychotics alone in social cognition. Sergi et al. (2007) evaluated social cognition during a double blind study comparing olanzapine, risperidone and haloperidol. They administered several social cognition measures (including tasks of emotion perception and social perception) at baseline, after 4 and 8 weeks of treatment. They developed a summary score of social cognition and observed no effect of antipsychotic treatment either within-group or between-groups on social cognition.

In relation to ToM, Savina and Beninger (2007) cross-sectionally compared groups of schizophrenic patients taking different antipsychotic drugs with healthy controls and concluded that patients treated with clozapine and with olanzapine had a better performance than patients taking risperidone or first generation antipsychotics. The clozapine and the olanzapine groups performed similarly as the controls. Mizrahi et al. (2007) evaluated the ToM of 17 drug-free psychotic patients (schizophrenia, schizophreniform and schizoaffective disorder) at baseline and every 2 weeks for 6 weeks, after initiating antipsychotic treatment (different second generation drugs) and observed an improvement in ToM performance. However, the authors could not exclude the influence of a practice effect due to the repetition of the ToM task and call attention to the lack of a placebo-control group. Recently, Pedersen et al. (2011), a randomized double-blind placebo controlled trial showed an improvement in ToM in patients treated with intranasal oxytocin for two weeks.

The influence of antipsychotic drugs in emotion recognition has been studied by several authors with positive (Cabral-Calderin et al. 2010, Fakra et al. 2009, Behere et al. 2009, Ibarrarán-Pernas et al. 2003) and negative results (Lewis and Garver 1995). The largest study of the impact of antipsychotic drugs on emotion recognition was conducted together with the CATIE study. This five-arm double-blind randomized study compared the effectiveness of olanzapine, risperidone, ziprasidone, quetiapine and perphenazine in chronic schizophrenic patients. Patients (n=873) were tested before randomization and two months after treatment. All antipsychotics showed a small, nonsignificant, improvement in emotion recognition; a lower baseline emotion recognition scores and higher baseline neurocognitive functioning predicted a better improvement in emotion recognition after two months of treatment (Penn et al. 2009). In a single dose, placebo controlled crossover trial, modafinil (200 mg) improved the recognition of sad faces in first episode psychosis (Scoriels et al 2011).

Littrell et al (2004) showed an improvement in social perception in patients treated with olanzapine. Treatment with oxytocin improved social perception in schizophrenia (Pedersen et al. 2011).

Considered together, these studies show some improvement of social cognition deficits with antipsychotic treatment. Nevertheless, not all studies were specifically designed to study this subject, and there are other methodological issues such as the use of different tests to evaluate social cognition. The issue of the learning effect by repeating the task after a few weeks is also not clearly addressed. It is not clear yet whether the influence of antipsychotics (or other drugs) on social cognition is direct or indirect, due to the improvement of psychopathology (especially positive symptoms).

3.3 Rehabilitation

Studies published in the last decades investigated the efficacy of psychosocial rehabilitation in medication-resistant positive symptoms, such as cognitive-behavioral therapy and social skills training. Residual symptom reduction is a major therapeutic goal. However, patients and their families in functional impairments at work, education, autonomy and socialization as a major concern. Difficulties in performing activities that require minimum critique of the real world is common in schizophrenia. Lack of social skills occurs even after a successful treatment of symptoms of the disease, presenting early and persisting all through life. (Granholm et al., 2009).

Around 2/3 of patients cannot achieve or sustain basic social roles such as a job, conjugal life, paternity/maternity and integration in the community. Rehabilitation approaches, such as social and vocational skills training and cognitive behavioral therapy aim at helping patients reduce impairments in social role functioning (Seth et al., 2010).

Social skills training aims at improving social impairments that are typical in schizophrenia, with strategies based on the application of principles of social learning. In the studies cited by Kurzban et al. (2010), several strategies have been implemented, such as vocational skills training, social training, self-care skills, communication skills and assertiveness training.

The studies in this area have indicated reduction of symptoms and improvement of functioning with different forms of cognitive therapies (Swerdlow, 2011), which can be computer-based or manual (Park et al., 2010). Generally speaking, cognitive therapies develop compensatory strategies for information learning and retrieval. They act in prefrontal areas of the brain, in charge of working memory and attention (Swerdlow, 2011).

3.3.1 Neuropsychological rehabilitation and social cognition

It is unlikely that interventions focused on neurocognition are sufficient to correct deficits in social cognition, since only around 40% of schizophrenics present specific cognitive deficits (Horan et al., 2009), although they may also present social inability (Horton & Silverstein, 2008).

Several studies relate social impairments to the high rate of relapse and low quality of life. However, recent attempts at associating cognitive training to social skills training have had partial success. Intense training of neurocognition improves cognitive deficits (attention, memory and executive functions, etc.), but does not automatically extend to social functioning (Choi & Kwon, 2006).

Non-pharmacological interventions aimed at cognitive deficits in schizophrenia are usually referred to as "cognitive remediation" or "cognitive training" (Galderisi et al., 2009). Cognitive remediation programs are rarely based on a clear theory, and quite often rely more on practice than on learning. Several approaches of cognitive training have been developed, such as computer-based repetitive cognitive exercises, or its pen and paper version, learning strategies for organization of information or adaptative strategies involving the environment and behavior, and strategies for learning, such as: instructions, positive reinforcement, etc. In a meta-analysis study on the efficacy of cognitive remediation therapy, significant cognitive improvement was verified, and a modest improvement in social functioning. Cognitive remediation in itself cannot address all the deficits and must be integrated with broader rehabilitation programs, including occupational therapy, professional counseling, self-care, among other therapeutic activities (Wykes et al., 2011, Patel et al., 2010).

The studies lean towards the development of strategies of cognitive rehabilitation, associating specific cognitive interventions with the domains of social cognition. The consensus battery of cognitive tests, MATRICS, identified social cognition as one of the seven critical cognitive domains for understanding schizophrenia (Horton & Silverstein, 2008). Some studies indicate that cognitive remediation improves cognitive performance, symptoms and psychosocial functioning. Other authors believe that cognitive remediation will be ineffective if it ignores social cognition and its components, and reviews suggest that the cognitive deficits are more associated with functional outcomes than to the psychiatric symptoms (Veltro et al., 2011).

Presently, there are two different types of intervention focused on developing social cognition. The first, called "target intervention", seeks to stimulate only one specific domain of social cognition. The second, named "broadbased interventions", consists of more eclectic and complex programs, which incorporate multiple domains. In three reviews, a significant improvement of the cognitive domain in question was found with both forms of intervention. However, it was not possible to claim a direct influence on social cognition. It was also noted that individuals with schizophrenia benefit from interventions which improve linguistic skills, especially those related to social cognition (Horton & Silverstein, 2008).

In a recent review of 19 studies and 692 patients, an effect size of 0.71 was found in emotion recognition in faces, small effect (d=0.46) in theory of the mind, and non-significant effect on social perception and attribution style. However, the generalization measures revealed a significant effect size in total symptoms (0.68) and functioning in the community. The effects of training in positive and negative symptoms were not significant (Horton & Silverstein, 2008). The limitation of training in social cognition in positive and negative symptoms described in this review may reflect the multidetermined nature of these domains of the disease, such as non-adherence to medication and family dysfunction. In turn, the verification of moderate effect size in general symptoms suggests an effective influence of general psychiatric symptom, such as depression and anxiety (Kurtz & Richardson, 2011).

According to Medalia & Choi (2009), several factors have influence over a positive treatment response for cognitive remediation training and social skills, such as training of the therapist, motivation of the patient, intensity and type of training and the base cognitive resources, which may be more or less preserved. The negative symptoms, however, may influence commitment to the work, relationship and treatment (Kurzban et al., 2010).

In most studies, the patients with the longest history of the disease were better prepared to make use of the social cognition intervention. The generalization of training in social cognition was also larger in young samples, with even more evident improvement when the treatment had longer duration and included prescribed medication (Kurtz & Richardson, 2011).

Nowadays, a large number of approaches is available. However, rather than envisage an extended intervention program which will encompass all, health professionals should devise customized treatments, avoiding unrealistic expectations. The disorder is heterogeneous in nature and may go through many changes over time (Penn et al., 2008).

Studies (n=10)	Sample	Type of Intervention	Major Findings
Choi & Kwon, 2006	34 patients diagnozed with schizophrenia	Training in psychiatric rehabilitation standard plus social cognition enhancement training (SCET)	Some social cognition skills improved rapidly after 2 months of treatment; however, other skills only improved after 6 months of treatment
Penn et al., 2007	17 hospitalized patients diagnozed with schizophrenia	Social cognition and interaction training (SCIT)	The patients exhibited better emotion recognition, theory of mind and reduced tendency to hostility towards others
Horan et al., 2008	31 stabilized clinic patients diagnozed with schizophrenia	Program of training in social cognition	The participants of the social training group presented significant improvement in facial emotion recognition
Horton & Silverstein, 2008	34 deaf and 31 non deaf schizophrenic patients	Training of cognition and social cognition	Non-deaf subjects did better at social cognition tasks including linguistic skills Deaf subjects exhibited better results in social cognition tasks which included non-linguistics tasks; facial affect processing (FAP) and ToM were effective in non-deaf subjects FAP consists of a more efficient mediator in deaf subjects
Wykes et al., 2008	29 patients diagnozed with schizophrenia	Individualized cognitive rehabilitation	Improvement in memory, mental flexibility and planning Secondary improvement of symptoms, social contact and self-esteem
Galderisi et al., 2009	60 randomized patients diagnozed with schizophrenia	Structured leisure activities (SLA) and social skills and neurocognitive individualized training (SSANIT)	After 6 months of treatment, patients with SSANIT training did better in social and personal functioning than those who underwent only SLA.
Park et al., 2010	91 hospitalized patients diagnozed with schizophrenia	Social skills training with traditional role playing (SST-TR) and Social skillls training through virtual reality (SST-VR)	The SST-VR group showed more improvement in conversation skill assertiveness, when compared with the SST-TR group, but less in non-verbal skills.
Patel et al., 2010	85 randomized patients with schizophrenia	Standard Cognitive Remediation Therapy (CRT), plus self-care	Improvement of working memory in CRT
Sparks et al., 2010	30 patients with schizophrenia or schizoaffective disorder and 25 healthy controls	Social cognition training involving emotion recognition	Participants with schizophrenia kept the worst performance in identifying emotional states in tests of discrimination of emotions in faces, when compared with the healthy controls group
Veltro et al., 2011	24 individuals diagnozed with schizophrenia	Cognitive emotional rehabilitation (REC) *vs* Problem solving training (PST)	Both training methods were efficient in psychopathological measures and social functioning

Table 5. Programs of training in social cognition and neuropschological rehabilitation.

4. Conclusions and limitations

4.1 Conclusions

Social cognition is of great importance in human interaction, enabling the adaptation of behavior in a wide range of social contexts. Deficits in social cognition, including all of its domains, are observed along the course of schizophrenia, even in the early stages of the disorder. It results in significant functional impairment, hindering independent living. Deficits in social cognition are also observed in first degree relatives of patients with schizophrenia and in individuals with schizotypal characteristics.

Interventions aimed to improve social cognitive abilities, minimizing the impact of deficits on their socio-emotional functioning are increasingly necessary.

Pharmacological treatments, especially second generation antipsychotics, seem to improve neurocognitive performance. However, the effects of such drugs on social cognition are still unclear and more studies are required to clarify their impact on social cognition.

Cognitive rehabilitation, associated with pharmacological treatment, has shown to be effective in improving social cognition in schizophrenia. However, it is still not possible to determine whether such improvements are preserved after the discontinuation of the intervention. It is likewise unclear whether these improvements are generalized beyond the therapeutic environment.

4.2 Limitations

The diagnostic criteria used, both for schizophrenia and for other psychotic disorders, are still controversial. In studies involving ultra high risk populations, additionally to the difficulty to characterize the individuals, the duration of follow up can impair the results of the study, as for some individuals the period to convert to psychosis or any other mental disorder may be longer than the usual period of follow up in the studies (one to two years).

There is marked heterogeneity both in the size of the samples used and in the social cognitive tests applied, bringing difficulties to compare the studies.

The use one single test to measure a specific aspect of social cognition may not be sufficient to measure the degree of impairment in social cognition, since an individual may show good performance in easier tasks (eg., emotion recognition in faces), but exhibit deficits in the ability to discriminate more complex kinds of social information (eg., emotion recognition in dynamic scenes or in prosody).

Impairments in neurocognition are well described in schizophrenia and may impair the accurate evaluation of social cognition, since some of its domains depend upon the good functioning of basic cognitive functions. It is not clear how neurocognition, social cognition and symptom domains interact with each other.

With respect to interventions, the studies do not clearly discuss learning effects of multiple applications of the tests in the same patients. The outcome may be influenced not only by the intervention, but also by the clinical condition of the patient.

5. References

Aakre, J.M.; Seghers J.P.; St-Hilaire A. & Docherty, N. (2009). Attributional style in delusional patients: a comparison of remitted paranoid, remitted nonparanoid, and current paranoid patients with nonpsychiatric controls. *Schizophrenia Bulletin*. Vol. 35, (September 2009), pp. 994-1002

Achim A.M.; Ouellet, R.; Roy, M.A. & Jackson, P.L. (2010). Assessment of empathy in first-episode psychosis and meta-analytic comparison with previous studies in schizophrenia. *Psychiatry Research*. (December 2010). [Epub ahead of print]

Addington, J. (2004). The diagnosis and assessment of individuals prodromal for schizophrenic psychosis. *CNS Spectrums*. Vol. 9, No 8. (August 2004), pp.588-94

Addington, J.; Penn, D.; Woods, S.W.; Addington, D. & Perkins, D.O. (2008). Facial affect recognition in individuals at clinical high risk for psychosis. *The British journal of psychiatry : the journal of mental science*. Vol. 192, No 1, (January 2008), pp. 67–68

Addington, J.; Saeedi, H. & Addington, D. (2006). Facial affect recognition: a mediator between cognitive and social functioning in psychosis? *Schizophrenia Research*. Vol. 85, No 1-3, (July 2006), pp. 142–50.

Adolphs R.; Tranel D.; Damasio H. & Damasio A. (1994). Impaired recognition of emotion in facial expressions following bilateral damage to the human amygdala. *Nature*, Vol.372, (1994), pp. 669-672.

Adolphs, R. (2001). The neurobiology of social cognition. *Current Opinion in Neurobiology*, Vol.11, (2001), pp. 231-239

Amminger, G.P.; Schäfer, M.R.; Papageorgiou, K.; Klier, C.M.; Schlögelhofer, M.; Mossaheb, N.; An, S.K.; Kang, J.I.; Park, J.Y.; Kim, K.R.; Lee, S.Y.& Lee, E. (2010). Attribution bias in ultra-high risk for psychosis and first-episode schizophrenia. *Schizophrenia Research*. Vol. 118, No 1-3, (May 2010), pp. 54-61.

Barch D.M. (2010). Pharmacological strategies for enhancing cognition in schizophrenia. (2010). *Current Top Behavior Neuroscience*. (january 2010), pp. 43-96

Bechara, A.; Damasio, H;, & Damasio, A. (2003). Role of the amygdala in decision-making. *Annals of the New York Academy of Sciences*, Vol.985, (2003), pp. 359-369

Behere, R.V.; Venkatasubramanian, G; Arasappa, R.; Reddy, N. & Gangadhar, B.N. (2009). Effect of risperidone on emotion recognition deficits in antipsychotic-naïve schizophrenia: a short-term follow-up study. *Schizophrenia Research*. Vol. 113, No 1, (August 2009), pp. 72-6

Bentall, R.P.; Corcoran, R.; Howard, R.; Blackwood, N. & Kinderman, P. (2001). Persecutory delusions: a review and theoretical integration. *Clinical Psychology Review*. Vol. 21, No 8, (November 2001), pp. 1143-92

Bertrand, M.C.; Sutton, H.; Achim, A.M.; Malla, A.K. & Lepage, M. (2007). Social cognitive impairments in first episode psychosis. *Schizophrenia Research*. Vol. 95, No 1-3, (September 2007), pp. 24-33

Bonshtein, U. (2006). Theory of mind in schizophrenia. *Harefuah*. Vol. 145, No 12, (December 2006), pp. 926-931, 939.

Bora, E. (2009). Theory of mind in schizophrenia spectrum disorders. *Turkish Journal of Psychiatry*. Vol. 20, No 3, (2009), pp. 269-81

Bora, E.; Yucel, M. & Pantelis, C. (2009). Theory of mind impairment in schizophrenia: meta-analysis. *Schizophrenia Research.* Vol. 109, No 1-3, (February 2009), pp. 1-9

Brown, L.A. & Cohen, A.S. (2010). Facial emotion recognition in schizotypy: the role of accuracy and social cognitive bias. *Journal of the International Neuropsychological Society.* Vol.16, No 3, (May, 2010), pp. 474-83

Brüne, M. & Brüne-Cohrs, U. (2006). Theory of mind - evolution, ontogeny, brain mechanisms and psychopathology. *Neuroscience and Biobehavioral Reviews.* Vol.30, (2006), pp. 437-455.

Brüne, M. (2005). Theory of mind" in schizophrenia: a review of the literature. *Schizophrenia Bulletin.* Vol. 3, No 1, (January 2005), pp. 21-42

Cabral-Calderin, Y. & Mendoza-Quiñones R.,; Garcia, A.; Caballero, A.; Dominguez, M.; Reyes, M.M. (2010). Effect of quetiapine treatment on facial emotion recognition deficits in schizophrenia patients. *Schizophrenia Research.* Vol. 119, No 1-3, (april 2010), pp. 275-6

Choi, K. & Kwon, J. (2006). Social Cognition Enhancement Training for Schizophrenia: A Preliminary Randomized Controlled Trial. *Community Mental Health Journal.* Vol. 42, No 2, (April 2006), pp. 177-187

Chung, Y.S.; Kang, D.H.; Shin, N.Y.; Yoo, S.Y. & Kwon, J.S. (2008). Deficit of theory of mind in individuals at ultra-high-risk for schizophrenia. Schizophr Research. Vol. 99, No 1-3, (February 2008), pp. 111-8

Couture S.M.; Penn D.L. & Roberts D.L. (2006). The functional significance of social cognition in schizophrenia: a review. *Schizophrenia Bulletin,* Vol.32, No.S1, (2006), pp. S44-S63.

Couture, S.M.; Penn, D.L.; Addington, J.; Woods, S.W. & Perkins, D.O. (2008). Assessment of social judgments and complex mental states in the early phases of psychosis. *Schizophrenia Research,* Vol.100, No.1-3, (March 2008), pp. 237-241

Del Prette, Z.A.P. & Del Prette, A. (2009). Psicologia das Habilidades Sociais: terapia, educação e trabalho. pp. 37-38. Editora Vozes, ISBN 978-85-326-2142-9, Rio de Janeiro.

Diez-Alegría, C.; Vázquez, C.; Nieto-Moreno, M.; Valiente, C. & Fuentenebro F. (2006). Personalizing and externalizing biases in deluded and depressed patients: are attributional biases a stable and specific characteristic of delusions? (2006). *Journal Clinical Psychological.* Vol. 45, No 4, (November 2006), pp. 531-44

Eack, S.M.; Mermon, D.E.; Montrose, D.M.; Miewald, J.; Gur, R.E.; Gur, R.C.; Sweeney, J.A. & Edwards, J., Pattison, P.E.; Jackson, H.J. & Wales, R.J. (2001). Facial affect and affective prosody recognition in first-episode schizophrenia. Schizophrenia Research. Vol. 30, No 48, 2-3, (March 2001), pp. 235-53

Emery N. & Amaral D. (2000). The role of the amygdala in primate social cognition. in R. Lane & L. Nadel (Orgs.), *Cognitive neurosciencie of emotion,* pp. 570-600, Oxford: Oxford University Press.

Emery, N.J & Clayton, N.S. (2009). Comparative social cognition. *Annual review of psychology.* Vol. 60, No 87, (2009), pp. 87-113

Erol, A.; Mete, L.; Sonmez, I. & Unal, E.K. (2010). Facial emotion recognition in patients with schizophrenia and their siblings. *Nordic Journal of Psychiatry*. Vol. 64, No 1, (2010), pp. 63-7

Fakra, E.; Salgado-Pineda, P.; Besnier, N; Azorin, J.M. & Blin, O. (2009). Risperidone versus haloperidol for facial affect recognition in schizophrenia: findings from a randomised study. *World Journal Biology Psychiatry*. Vol. 10, No 4, (January 2009), pp. 719-28

Fett, A-K.J.; Viechtbauerb, W. & Domingueza, M.G. (2011). The relationship between neurocognition and social cognition with functional outcomes in schizophrenia: A meta-analysis. *Neuroscience and Biobehavioral Reviews*. Vol. 35, (2011), pp. 573-588

Frommann, I.; Pukrop, R.; Brinkmeyer, J.; Bechdolf, A.; Ruhrmann, S.; Berning, J.; Decker, P.; Riedel, M.; Möller, H.J.; Wölwer, W.; Gaebel, W.; Klosterkötter, J.; Maier, W. & Wagner, M. (2011). Neuropsychological Profiles in Different At-Risk States of Psychosis: Executive Control Impairment in the Early and Additional Memory Dysfunction in the Late-Prodromal State. *Schizophrenia Bulletin*. Vol. 37, No 4, (July 2011), pp. 861-73.

Fuentes, D.; Lunardi, L.L.; Malloy-Diniz, L. F. & Rocca, C.C. de A. (2010). Cap. 15. Reconhecimento de Emoções, in Avaliação Neuropsicológica. Malloy-Diniz, L.F.; Fuentes, D.; Mattos, P.; Abreu, N. & Cols. pp. 169-174. Editora Artmed, ISBN 978-85-363-2210-0, Porto Alegre.

Galderisi, S.; Piegari, G.; Mucci, A.; Acerra, A.; Luciano, L.; Rabasca, A.F.; Santucci, F.; Valente, A.; Volpe M.; Gibson, C.M.; Penn, D.L.; Prinstein, M.J.; Perkins, D.O. & Belger, A. (2010). Social skill and social cognition in adolescents at genetic risk for psychosis. *Schizophrenia Research*. Vol. 122, No 1-3, (September 2010), pp. 179–184

Granholm, E; Ben-zeev, Dror. & Link, P.C. (2009). Social desinterest attitudes and group cognitive-behavioral social skills training for functional disability in schizophrenia. (2009). *Schizophrenia Bulletin*. Vol. 35, No 5, (July 2009), pp. 874-883

Green, M.F.; Bearden, C.E.; Cannon, T.D.; Fiske, A.P.; Hellemann, G.S.; Horan, W.P.; Kee, K.; Kern, R.S.; Lee, J.; Sergi, M.J.; Subotnik, K.L.; Sugar, C.A.; Ventura, J.; Yee, C.M. & Nuechterlein, K.H. (2011). Social Cognition in Schizophrenia, Part 1: Performance Across Phase of Illness. *Schizophrenia Bulletin*. 2011 (Feb 23). [Epub ahead of print]

Horan, W.P.; Kern, R.S.; Shokat-Fadai, K.; Sergi, M.J.; Wynn, J.K. & Green, M.F. (2008). Social cognitive skills training in schizophrenia: an initial efficacy study of stabilized outpatients. *Schizophrenia Research*. Vol. 107, No 1, (January 2009), pp. 47-54

Horton, H.K. & Silverstein, S.M.(2008). Social cognition as a mediator of cognition and outcome among deaf and hearing people with schizophrenia. *Schizophrenia Research*. Vol. 105, (August 2008), pp. 125-137

Ibarrarán-Pernas, G.Y.; Guevara, M.A.; Cerdán, L.F. & Ramos-Loyo, J. (2003). Olanzapine effects on emotional recognition in treatment refractory schizophrenics. *Actas Esp Psiquiatry*. Vol. 31, No 5, (October 2003), pp. 256-62

Janssen, I.; Versmissen, D.; Campo, J.A.; Myin-Germeys, I.; van Os J & Krabbendam, L. (2006). Attribution style and psychosis: evidence for an externalizing bias in patients but not in individuals at high risk. *Psychological Medicine*. Vol. 36, No 6, (June 2006), pp. 771-8

Kim, H.S.; Shin, N.Y.; Choi, J.S.; Jung, M.H.; Jang, J.H.; Kang, D.H. & Kwon, J.S. (2010). Processing of facial configuration in individuals at ultra-high risk for schizophrenia. *Schizophrenia Research.* Vol. 118, No 1-3, (May 2010), pp. 81-7

Keshavan, M.S. (2010). Social cognition deficits among individuals at familial high risk for schizophrenia. *Schizophrenia Bulletin*. Vol. 36, No 6, (November 2010), pp.1081-8

Koelkebeck, K.; Pedersen, A.; Suslow, T.; Kueppers, K.A.; Arolt, V. & Ohrmann, P. (2010). Theory of Mind in first-episode schizophrenia patients: correlations with cognition and personality traits. *Schizophrenia Research.* Vol. 119, No 1-3, (June 2010), pp. 115-23

Kohler, C.G.; Turner, T.H.; Gur, R.E. & Gur, R.C. (2004). Recognition of facial emotions in neuropsychiatric disorders. CNS *Spectrums*. Vol.9, No. 4, (2004), pp. 267-275

Kohler, C.G.; Martin, E.A.; Kujawski, E.; Bilker, W.; Gur R.E. & Gur, R.C. (2007). No effect of donepezil on neurocognition and social cognition in young persons with stable schizophrenia. *Cognition Neuropsychiatry*. Vol. 12, No 5, (September 2007), pp. 412-21

Kohler, C.G.; Walker, J. B.; Martin, E.A.; Healey, K.M.; & Moberg, P.J. (2010). Facial emotion perception in schizophrenia: a meta-analytic review. *Schizophrenia Bulletin*. Vol. 36, No 5, (September 2010), pp. 1009-19

Kraemer, H.C. & Kupfer, D.J.(2005). Size of treatment effects and their importance to clinical research and practice. *Biological Psychiatry*. Vol. 59, No 11, (June 2006), pp. 990-6

Krstev, H.; Jackson, H. & Maude, D. (1999). An investigation of attributional style in first-episode psychosis. *British Journal of Social and Clinical Psychology*. Pt 2, (June 1999), pp. 181-94

Krueger F.; Barbey A.K. & Grafman J. (2009). The medial prefrontal cortex mediates social event knowledge. Trends Cognition Science. Vol.13, (Febrary 2009), [Epub ahead of print]

Kurtz, M.M. & Richardson, C.L. (2011). Social Cognitive Training for Schizophrenia: A Meta-Analytic Investigation of Controlled Research. *Schizophrenia Bulletin.* Vol.27, (April 2011), pp. 1-13.

Kurzban, S.; Davis, L. & Breke, J.S. (2010). Vocational, Social, and Cognitive Rehabilitation for individuals diagnosed with schizophrenia: a review of recent research and trends. *Current Psychiatry Rep*. Vol. 12, (June 2010), pp. 345-355

Lewis, S.F. & Garver, D.L. (1995). Treatment and diagnostic subtype in facial affect recognition in schizophrenia. *Journal Psychiatry Research.* Vol. 29, No 1, (January-February 1995), pp. 5-11

Li, H.; Chan, R.C.; Zhao, Q.; Hong, X. & Gong, Q.Y. (2010). Facial emotion perception in Chinese patients with schizophrenia and non-psychotic first-degree relatives. *Progress in Neuro-Psychopharmacology and Biological Psychiatry*. Vol. 34, No 2, (March 2010), pp. 393-400.

Littrell, K.H.; Petty, R.G.; Hilligoss, N.M.; Kirshner, C.D. & Johnson, C.G. (2004). Improvement in social cognition in patients with schizophrenia associated with treatment with olanzapine. *Schizophrenia Research.* Vol. 66, No 2-3, (February 2004), pp. 201-2

Mastantuono, P. & Maj, M.(2010). Social skills and neurocognitive individualized training in schizophrenia: comparison with structured leisure activities. *Europe Archiment Psychiatry Clinical Neuroscience*. Vol. 260, No 4, (October 2009), pp. 305-15

Marwick, K. & Hall, J. (2008). Social cognition in schizophrenia: a review of face processing. *British Medical Bulletin*. Vol. 88, No 1, (2008), pp. 43-58

Medalia, A. & Choi, J. (2009). Cogntive remediation in schizophrenia. (2009). *Neuropsychological Reviews*. Vol. 19, No 3, (May 2009), pp. 353-364

McGorry, P.D.; Yung, A.R. & Phillips, L.J. (2003). The "close-in" or ultra high-risk model: a safe and effective strategy for research and clinical intervention in prepsychotic mental disorder. *Schizophrenia Bulletin*. Vol. 29, No 4, (2003), pp. 771-90

Mishara, A.L. & Goldberg, T.E. (2004). A meta-analysis and critical review of the effects of conventional neuroleptic treatment on cognition in schizophrenia: opening a closed book. *Biology Psychiatry*. Vol. 55, No 10, (May 2004), pp. 1013-22

Mizrahi R.; Addington, J.; Remington, G. & Kapur, S. Attribution style as a factor in psychosis and symptom resolution. (2008). *Schizophrenia Research*. Vol.104, No 1-3, (July 2008), pp. 220-7

Mizrahi R.; Korostil, M.; Starkstein, S.E.; Zipursky, R.B. & Kapur, S. The effect of antipsychotic treatment on Theory of Mind. (2007). *Psychological Medicine*. Vol. 37, No 4, (November 2006), pp. 595-601

Mizrahi, R.; Addington, J.; Remington, G. & Kapur, S. (2008). Attribution style as a factor in psychosis and symptom resolution. *Schizophrenia Bulletin*. Vol. 104, No 1-3, (September 2008), pp. 220-7

Monteiro, L.C. & Louzã, M.R. (2010). Cap. 14. Cognição Social, in *Avaliação Neuropsicológica*. Malloy-Diniz, L.F.; Fuentes, D.; Mattos, P.; Abreu, N. & Cols. pp. 162-168. Editora Artmed, ISBN 978-85-363-2210-0, Porto Alegre.

Monteiro, L.C.; Queiroz, F.P. & Rössler, W. (2010). Cap. 16. Teoria da Mente, in *Avaliação Neuropsicológica*. Malloy-Diniz, L.F.; Fuentes, D.; Mattos, P.; Abreu, N. & Cols. pp. 175-182. Editora Artmed, ISBN 978-85-363-2210-0, Porto Alegre

Morris, R.W.; Weickert, C.S. & Loughland, C.M. (2009). Emotional face processing in schizophrenia. *Current Opinion in Psychiatry*. Vol. 22, No 2, (March 2009), pp. 140-6

Niendam, T.A.; Bearden, C.E.; Zinberg, J.; Johnson, J.K.; O'Brien, M. & Cannon, T.D. (2007). The course of neurocognition and social functioning in individuals at ultra high risk for psychosis. *Schizophrenia Bulletin*. Vol. 33, No 3, (May, 2007), pp. 772-81

Ochsner, K.N. Current directions in social cognitive neuroscience. *Current Opinion in Neurobiology*, Vol.14, No. 2, (2004), pp. 254-258

Park, K.; Ku, J.; Choi, S.; Jang, H.; Park, J.; Kim, S.I. & Kim, J. (2011). A virtual reality application in role-plays of social skills training for schizophrenia: a randomized, controlled trial. *Psychiatry Research*. (April 2011), pp. 1-7

Patel, A.; Knapp, M.; Romeo, R.; Reeder, C.; Matthiasson, P.; Everitt, B. & Wykes, T. (2010). Cognitive remediation therapy in schizophrenia: cost-effectiveness analysis. *Schizophrenia Research*. Vol. 120, No 3, (January 2010), pp. 217-24

Pedersen, C.A.; Gibson, C.M.; Rau, S.W.; Salimi, K.; Smedley, K.L.; Casey, R.L.; Leserman, J.; Jarskog, L.F. & Penn, D.L. (2011). Intranasal oxytocin reduces psychotic symptoms and improves Theory of Mind and social perception in schizophrenia. *Schizophrenia Research*. (August 2011), [ahead of print]

Penn, D.L.; Sanna, L.J. & Roberts, D.L. (2008). Social cognition in schizophrenia: an overview. *Schizophrenia Bulletin*, Vol.34, No. 3, pp. 408-411

Penn, D.L.; Keefe, R.S.; Davis, S.M.; Meyer, P.S.; Perkins, D.O.; Losardo, D. & Lieberman, J.A. (2009). The effects of antipsychotic medications on emotion perception in patients with chronic schizophrenia in the CATIE trial. *Schizophrenia Research*. Vol. 115, No 1, (September 2009), pp. 17-23

Penn, D.L.; Roberts, D.L.; Combs, D. & Sterne, A. (2007). The development of the social cognition and interction training program for schizophrenia spectrum disorders. *Psichiatric services*. Vol. 58, No 4, (April 2007), pp. 449-451

Penn, D.L.; Sanna, L.J. & Roberts, D.L. (2008). Social cognition in schizophrenia: an overview. *Schizophrenia bulletin*. Vol. 34, No 3, (March 2008), pp. 408-11

Penn, D.L.; Corrigan, P.W.; Bentall, R.P. & Racenstein, J.M. (1997). Social cognition in schizophrenia. *Psychological Bulletin*, Vol.121, No. 1, (1997), pp. 114-132.

Peters E. & Garety P. Cognitive functioning in delusions: a longitudinal analysis. *Behavior Research Therapy*. Vol. 44, No 4, (April 2006), pp. 481-514

Pinkham, A.E.; Penn, D.L.; Perkins, D.O.; Graham, K.A. & Siegel, M. (2007). Emotion perception and social skill over the course of psychosis: a comparison of individuals "at-risk" for psychosis and individuals with early and chronic schizophrenia spectrum illness. *Cognitive Neuropsychiatry*. Vol. 12, No3, (May. 2007), pp. 198-212

Reed, S. I. (2008). First-episode psychosis: A literature review. *International Journal of Mental Health Nursing*. Vol. 17, (2008), pp. 85–91

Rocca, C.C.A.; Polisel, A.F.; Mattos, K.M.G. & Silva, M.C.F. (2010). Cap. 17. Habilidades Sociais, in *Avaliação Neuropsicológica*. Malloy-Diniz, L.F.; Fuentes, D.; Mattos, P.; Abreu, N. & Cols. pp. 183-197. Editora Artmed, ISBN 978-85-363-2210-0, Porto Alegre

Sachs, G.; Steger-Wuchse, D.; Kryspin-Exner, I.; Gur, R.C. & Katschnig, H. (2004). Facial recognition deficits and cognition in schizophrenia. Schizophrenia Research. Vol. 1, No 68-1, (May, 2004), pp.27-35

Satpute A.B. & Lieberman M.D. (2006). Integrating automatic and controlled processes into neurocognitive models of social cognition. *Brain Research*. Vol.1079, (2006), pp. 86-97

Savina I. & Beninger, R.J. Schizophrenic patients treated with clozapine or olanzapine perform better on theory of mind tasks than those treated with risperidone or typical antipsychotic medications. (2007). *Schizophrenia Research*. Vol. 94, No 1-3, (June 2007), pp. 128-38

Scoriels, L.; Barnett, J.H.; Murray, G.K.; Cherukuru, S.; Fielding, M.; Cheng, F.; Lennox, BR.; Sahakian, B.J. & Jones, P.B. (2010). Effects of modafinil on emotional processing in first episode psychosis. *Biological Psychiatry*. Vol. 69, No 5, (December 2011), pp. 457-64

Seligman, M. E. P.; Nolen-Hoeksema, S.; Thornton, N. & Thornton, K. M. (1990). Explanatory style as a mechanism of disappointing athletic performance. *Psychological Science*. Vol.1, (1990), pp.143-146

Sergi, M.J.; Green, M.F.; Widmark, C.; Reist, C.; Erhart, S.; Braff, D.L.; Kee, K.S.; Marder, S.R. & Mintz, J. (2007). Social cognition and neurocognition: effects of risperidone, olanzapine, and haloperidol. *American Journal Psychiatry*. Vol. 164, No 10, (October 2007), pp. 1585-92

So, S.H.; Garety, P.A.; Peters, E.R. & Kapur, S. (2010). Do antipsychotics improve reasoning biases? A review. *Psychossomatic Medicine*. Vol. 72, No 7, (July 2010), pp. 681-93

Sparks A.; McDonald, S.; Lino, B.; O'Donnell, M. & Green, M.J. (2010). Social Cognition, empathy and functional outcome in schizophrenia. *Schizophrenia Research*. Vol. 122, (May 2010), pp. 172-8

Sprong, M.; Schothorst, P.; Vos E.; Hox, J. & van Engeland, H. (2007). Theory of mind in schizophrenia: meta-analysis. The British journal of psychiatry : the journal of mental science. Vol. 191 (Jul. 2007), pp. 5-13.

Swerdlow, N.R. (2011). Are we studying and treating schizophrenia correctly? *Schizophrenia Research*. Vol. 130, No 1-3, (June 2011), pp. 1-10

The British journal of psychiatry: the journal of mental science. Vol. 109, No 1-3, (April 2009), pp. 1-9

Thompson, A.D.; Bartholomeusz, C. & Yung, A.R. (2011). Social cognition deficits and the 'ultra high risk' for psychosis population: a review of literature. *Early Intervention in Psychiatry*. Vol. 5, No 3, (Aug. 2011), pp. 192-202

Thornton, A.E.; Van Snellenberg, J.X.; Sepehry, A.A. & Honer, W. (2005). The impact of atypical antipsychotic medications on long-term memory dysfunction in schizophrenia spectrum disorder: a quantitative review. *Journal Psychopharmacological*. Vol. 20, No 3, (September 2005), pp. 335-46

Tonelli, H. A.; Alvarez, C. E. & Silva, A. A. (2009). Esquizotipia, "Teoria da Mente" habilidades e vulnerabilidade à psicose: uma revisão sistemática. *Revista Psiquiatria Clínica*. Vol. 36, No 6, (2009), pp.229-239. ISSN 0101-6083

Veltro, F.; Mazza, M.; Venditelli, N.; Alberti, M.; Casacchia, M. & Roncone, R. (2011). A comparison of the effectiveness of problem solving training and of cognitive-emotional rehabilitation on neurocognition, social cognition and social functioning in people with schizophrenia. *Clinical Practice e Epidemiology in Mental Health*, No 7, (July 2011), pp. 123-132

Woodward, N.D.; Purdon, S.E.; Meltzer, H.Y. & Zald, D.H. (2005). A meta-analysis of neuropsychological change to clozapine, olanzapine, quetiapine, and risperidone in schizophrenia. *International Jounal Neuropsychopharmacological*. Vol. 8, No 3, (March 2005), pp. 457-72

Werneck-Rohrer. S.; Nelson, B. & McGorry, P.D. (2011). Emotion Recognition in Individuals at Clinical High-Risk for Schizophrenia. *Schizophrenia Bulletin*. (March 2011), pp. 21

Wykes, T.; Huddy, V.; Cellard, C.C.; McGurk, S.R. & Czoborp. (2011). A meta-analysis of cognitive remediation for schizophrenia: methodoly and effect sizes. *American Journal Psychiatry*. Vol. 168, (May 2011), pp. 472-485

Wykes, T.; Newton, E; Landau, S.; Rice, C.; Thompson, N. & Frangou, S.(2008). Cognitive remediation therapy (CRT) for young early onset patients with schizophrenia: An exploratory randomized controlled trial. *Schizophrenia Research*. Vol. 94, No 1-3, (November 2008), pp. 221-3

4

Cognitive Remediation Therapy (CRT): Improving Neurocognition and Functioning in Schizophrenia

Rafael Penadés and Rosa Catalán
Institute of Clinical Neurosciences, Hospital Clínic de Barcelona, Department of Psychiatry and Psychobiology, University of Barcelona, IDIBAPS-CIBERSAM, Barcelona
Spain

1. Introduction

Schizophrenia is generally viewed as a chronic disorder characterized by psychotic symptoms and relatively stable neurocognitive and interpersonal deficits. According to the revised fourth edition of the Diagnostic and Statistical Manual of Mental Disorders (DSM-IV-TR), to be diagnosed with schizophrenia, three diagnostic criteria must be met (APA 2000):

1. Characteristic symptoms: Two or more of the following, each present for much of the time during a one-month period (or less, if symptoms remitted with treatment).
   - Delusions
   - Hallucinations
   - Disorganized speech, which is a manifestation of formal thought disorder
   - Grossly disorganized behaviour (e.g. dressing inappropriately, crying frequently) or catatonic behaviour
   - Negative symptoms: Blunted affect (lack or decline in emotional response), alogia (lack or decline in speech), or avolition (lack or decline in motivation)

If the delusions are judged to be bizarre, or hallucinations consist of hearing one voice participating in a running commentary of the patient's actions or of hearing two or more voices conversing with each other, only that symptom is required above. The speech disorganization criterion is only met if it is severe enough to substantially impair communication.

2. Social or occupational dysfunction: For a significant portion of the time since the onset of the disturbance, one or more major areas of functioning such as work, interpersonal relations, or self-care, are markedly below the level achieved prior to the onset.
3. Significant duration: Continuous signs of the disturbance persist for at least six months. This six-month period must include at least one month of symptoms (or less, if symptoms remitted with treatment).

The primary treatment of schizophrenia is antipsychotic medications, often in combination with psychological and social supports. Antipsychotic medication has made it possible to reduce psychotic symptoms and to prevent relapses, but is it expected that antipsychotic medication could, one day, improve cognition. Frequently, residual cognitive impairments stand as impediments to full recovery from schizophrenia (Bell and Berson, 2001). A number of psychosocial interventions may be useful in the treatment of schizophrenia including: family therapy, supported employment, cognitive remediation, skills training, cognitive behavioural therapy (CBT), token economic interventions, and psychosocial interventions for substance use and weight management. Cognitive Remediation Therapy (CRT) is a promising new treatment designed to improve neurocognitive abilities such as attention, memory and executive functioning. A large body of data on the efficacy of cognitive remediation therapy has been produced, and a number of meta-analyses have shown moderate to large effects on cognitive outcomes. However, experts in the field claim that CRT should not only enhance cognition but also that the improvement in cognition will affect community functioning. Consequently, clinicians are now increasingly concerned with identifying appropriate cognitive targets and ways of promoting secondary improvements in functioning.

2. Neuropsychology in schizophrenia

Current neuropsychological models of schizophrenia assert that cognitive impairments found in patients are simply the expression of some abnormalities in brain functioning. These abnormalities are found mainly in the frontal lobe and lead to a reduced capacity to activate frontal areas when faced with a cognitive challenge. In addition, multiple connectivity abnormalities between different brain regions have also been described. More specifically, it seems that the neural circuits interconnecting the limbic, the temporal and the frontal lobe are irregularly connected (Barch 2005). This model has received considerable support in empirical studies from various disciplines including neuroimaging, electrophysiology, neuropsychology and cognitive psychology (Andreasen, 1997). In an excellent review, Shenton et al. (2001) described the anatomical abnormalities that have been replicated most consistently in schizophrenia research: cavum septum pellucidum (92%), amygdala or hippocampus (74%), lateral ventricles (73%), basal ganglia (68%), superior temporal gyrus (67%), corpus callosum (63%), temporal lobe (61%), thalamus (42%), cerebellum (31%) and brain volume (22%). Nevertheless, the proposed model goes beyond the direct relationship between anatomical abnormalities and neurocognitive impairments. None of the aforementioned brain areas work in isolation. Rather, they work together as a part of different cortico-subcortical circuits linking the frontal cortex with other brain regions, such as the limbic system, basal ganglia and thalamus (Pearlson et al., 1996). This type of "disconnection" between brain areas would involve defective processing of information and be expressed as cognitive impairment (Weinberger & Lipska 1995).

Thus, due to the heterogeneity of the causes of cognitive impairments, it is more common to find different cognitive profiles with selective cognitive impairments than homogeneous, generalized cognitive impairment. Different sorts of dysfunctions have been described in various domains such as attention, vigilance, verbal memory and working memory. Additionally, patients with schizophrenia present serious difficulties in executive functioning: inflexibility, poor self-monitoring, lack of planning, and passive performance due to a lack of cognitive strategies. Problems with motor skills and difficulty in suppressing or inhibiting inappropriate responses are also present. Heinrichs & Zakzanis (1998) conducted a meta-analysis of more than 200 studies and found that between 60-80%

of patients with schizophrenia have neurocognitive impairments that can be classified as moderate or severe. However, it was not possible to find a unique cognitive profile for all patients. Various combinations of impairments including attention, working memory, verbal or visual learning, psychomotor speed and executive function were described (Table 1). Therefore, heterogeneity across all possible conceivable neurocognitive domains is perhaps what best describes the pattern of neurocognitive impairment in schizophrenia. Nevertheless, although the neuropsychological assessment of a patient diagnosed with schizophrenia may reflect an impaired profile through a number of domains such as attention, vigilance, verbal memory and working memory, the presence of attention and executive impairments are the common feature.

MILD IMPAIRMENT 0.5-1 SD below the mean	MODERATE IMPAIRMENT 1-2 SD below the mean	SEVERE IMPAIRMENT <2 SD below the mean
Perceptual skills	Verbal memory	Executive function
Speed processing	Working memory	Verbal fluency
Recognition memory	Recall memory	Verbal learning
Naming	Visuo-motor skills	Motor speed
General Intelligence	Distractibility	Vigilance

Table 1. The severity of cognitive impairments in schizophrenia.

3. Relevance of neurocognition in schizophrenia

Neurocognitive impairments in schizophrenia are not trivial because they are consistently associated with low social functioning and worse outcomes. Up to 60% of the variance in social functioning seems to be explained by neurocognitive variables. Performance in tests of attention, working memory, verbal memory, psychomotor speed and executive functions have been shown to be selectively related to different aspects of psychosocial functioning ranging from the level of independence in daily living skills, work performance and use of psychiatric services to the ability to learn new skills. Green (1996) conducted an important meta-analytic study attempting to test the aforementioned putative relationship between neurocognition and functioning. A positive and significant relationship between cognition and functioning was established through the meta-analysis and the various cognitive domains showed significant correlations. More specifically, verbal memory acted as the most robust predictor of functioning including social functioning, social problem solving and learning new skills. This close relationship has been replicated in other studies. Additionally, in former studies other variables including attention, processing speed and executive functions also proved to be strongly related to psychosocial functioning (Table 2). The presence of impairments in both verbal memory and attention span would affect the ability to acquire social skills and might be associated with considerable social dysfunctions.

	Vigilance	Working Memory	Verbal Memory	Executive Function
Social Functioning	+		+	
Vocational Functioning	+	+	+	+
Autonomy		+	+	+

Table 2. Relationship between cognitive performance and functioning.

Furthermore, some specific neuropsychological tests such as the Wisconsin Card Sorting Test (WCST) can be useful in the prediction of concrete aspects of functioning such as work performance (Lysaker et al. 1996). This test has shown an acceptable level of prediction regarding work performance in patients with schizophrenia. Thus, bad performance on the WCST is associated with fewer working hours in a competitive job, increased likeliness of emergent symptoms during the workday and the possibility of new hospital admissions. McGurk & Melter (2003) have pointed to neurocognitive aspects as the most important factors to be taken into account when attempting to return to work. Finally, it should be emphasised that cognitive impairments may interact with negative symptoms. Even further, some authors suggest that the combination of problems, negative symptoms and cognitive dysfunction would themselves generate pervasive social dysfunction. This is especially pernicious as some negative symptoms would prevent the patient being involved in rehabilitation programs.

4. Evidence-based treatments

Initially, neuropsychological rehabilitation programs used in brain injury were the best option for treating cognitive impairment in patients with schizophrenia. Other interventions used in degenerative processes and elderly people were also tried. Nowadays, this practice would not be considered appropriate because cognitive rehabilitation in schizophrenia has its own peculiarities. Therefore, it is highly advisable to use specific interventions, especially those that have been proven to be effective in controlled studies. Various approaches seem to be efficacious and effective alternatives. Interestingly, all these cognitive remediation therapies for schizophrenia have in common that they are types of behavioural training that aim to improve cognitive processes (attention, memory, executive function, social cognition or metacognition) with the goal of durability and generalization (Crew, 2010). Another important feature of evidence-based cognitive remediation therapies is the aim of enhancing cognition with the expectation that improved cognition will affect community functioning.

4.1 Integrated Psychological Therapy (IPT)

Integrated Psychological Therapy for Schizophrenia (IPT) was probably the first therapy to include neurocognitive elements specially developed to be used with schizophrenia patients (Brenner et al., 1992). It was designed by Professor Hans Dieter Brenner and colleagues at the University of Bern in Switzerland. There are versions in German, English and Spanish, adapted by Professor Volker Roder. The IPT is a structured intervention program that prescribes steps for treating cognitive and behavioural dysfunctions (Roder et al. 2007). It comprises five modules, applied in the following order: cognitive differentiation, social perception, communication, social skills, and interpersonal problem solving (Table 3). Although the main objective is the treatment of neurocognitive disorders, it also includes psychosocial elements, such as social skills training designed to improve social behavior deficit. The duration of the intervention generally ranges between 8 and 12 months although it is not established a priori and depends on the needs and progress of the participants during the course of treatment. It is a group therapy and is implemented twice a week for between 45 and 90 minutes. Ideally, group size is between four and eight participants. Support materials are very simple: a room, a blackboard, projector, paper, and pencils or pens. Learning techniques are frequently used such as token economy, discriminate learning, social reinforcement, modelling and shaping. Group dynamic techniques are also required including sharing, coaching, role playing, reformulation and positive connotation.

MODULES	TARGETS	INTERVENTION TECHNIQUES
Cognitive Differentiation	Attention Concept formation Abstraction	Card Sorting Verbal concept exercises
Social Perception	Social cognition	Slides depicting social situations Collecting information Interpretation and discussion Assigning a title
Verbal Communication	Communication skills	Literal repetition Paraphrasing W-Questions Topical questions Focused communication
Social Skills	Social Skills	Cognitive analysis Role-playing
Problem solving	Interpersonal problem solving	Problem solving technique Generalisation

Table 3. Modules of the Integrated Psychological Treatment (IPT).

The Cognitive Differentiation module seeks to improve attention (selective attention, focused attention, sustained attention, alternating attention, etc.) and also conceptualization skills (abstraction, concept formation, conceptual discrimination, etc.). The exercises consist of sorting cards; managing verbal concepts; elaborating definitions; managing words in different contextual meanings, and so on. The use of reinforcement is especially important in this part of the program to overcome motivational problems and negative symptoms. The Social Perception module seeks to improve the analysis and understanding of psychosocial information. This is neurocognitive work but focused on the social cognition processes. Different slides displaying social interaction situations are shown to the patients to be analyzed and interpreted. Each slide gives the opportunity for some analysis, coding, integration and understanding of social information. Therapists try to stimulate patients' abilities to discriminate between relevant and informative parts and the irrelevant stimuli. To achieve these targets, therapists use a variety of techniques including shaping, modelling and coaching. The Communication module targets relevant aspects of communication and interpersonal behavioural skills. It is designed to work with the three basic processes of language: listening, understanding and speaking. A series of verbal exercises are proposed in order to determine the effects of cognitive impairment on communication. These move from the literal repetition of sentences, formulation of questions and answers, to free communication exercises which gradually involve patients in interactive communication exercises. The Social Skills module aims to practice the necessary skills that enable patients to have satisfactory psychosocial functioning. The authors emphasize that learning through role-play requires memorization and analysis of social behaviour. Both processes may be altered as a consequence of cognitive impairments. Therapists encouraged the practice of these skills in real contexts to compensate for cognitive difficulties. Finally, the Problem Solving module brings the program to an end. The main objective is to increase the likelihood of solving the typical problems that appear in usual contexts. The intention is to allow the patient to be able to identify problems, to develop a rational attitude towards them and to focus on solutions rather than the problem itself so ultimately, fostering a thinking style that anticipates and takes into account the consequences of the chosen solutions. As is well known, all of these skills require a high degree of self-management that is not frequently found in patients suffering from executive dysfunction. A recent meta-analysis has confirmed the effectiveness of this therapy (Roder et al. 2006).

4.2 Cognitive Enhancement Therapy (CET)

The Cognitive Enhancement Therapy (CET) program was described by Hogarty & Flesher (1999 a, 1999 b). It was designed to be applied to patients with schizophrenia who show significant social and functional disability following pharmacological stabilization. CET has two complementary targets: neurocognitive rehabilitation and improvement of social cognition. It is intended that patients develop the cognitive and social skills that will be required for proper functioning in real interpersonal settings. It is primarily based on cognitive strategy instruction through computer tasks and group socialization experiences.

The program consists of two distinct parts: a neurocognitive training module and a social cognition module. Neurocognitive training is done individually and assisted with computer programs. It should be stressed that the exercises are done on the computer with the help of a peer and guided by a therapist. The social cognition training is done in groups through structured exercises and the practice of social interactions in real-life situations. Individual neurocognitive training is done through a series of exercises of increasing difficulty using computer programs on a PC. The training lasts about 60 hours and in each session performance on various tasks is discussed with another patient and the therapist who will carry out the necessary coaching. In terms of content, training is divided into attention, memory and problem-solving modules. Attention training is performed using computerized tasks from other programs such as the Orientation Remediation Module Ben-Yishay (1980) and the Bracy Computer Program (1987). Additionally, memory training aims to practice a number of skills that are supposed to improve memory performance. Categorization ability, use of abstract thinking and a flexible cognitive style on spatial and verbal tasks are all encouraged. Finally, improvement in problem-solving capacity is done through the practice of analytical thinking, planning, generation of alternatives and social intuition by reading clues.

The other component of the program is training in social cognition. This training is conducted in groups and aims to improve the cognitive skills required for effective interpersonal behaviour. Groups consist of 6 to 8 patients participating in 45 weekly sessions lasting one hour. Examples of the session topics are: understanding the others point of view, reading nonverbal signals or adjusting personal behaviour to the norms and rules of the social context. Group exercises are a way of generating real experiences to facilitate the learning of a variety of skills such as taking others' perspectives), interpreting contextual variables, solving potential social conflicts, and practicing emotion recognition, cognitive flexibility, abstract thinking and planning. The group exercises include categorization guidelines, construction of verbal messages, initiation and maintenance of a conversation, and extracting the central message from the opinion pages of a newspaper (the authors used the online version of USA Today). In other tasks, therapists encourage participants to interpret ambiguous scenes in interpersonal contexts in terms of social and emotional content. Participants are asked to interpret the intentions of various actors in a scene and to produce a written report highlighting the most relevant leading roles. This program was tested in a methodologically rigorous study, with a 2 year follow-up, and showed improvements in verbal memory, processing speed, social cognition and social adjustment (Hogarty et al. 2004).

4.3 Cognitive Remediation Therapy (CRT)

Initially developed in Australia by Ann Delahunty and reformulated by Til Wykes in the United Kingdom, this rehabilitation program aims to remediate cognitive impairments in schizophrenia patients by targeting executive functions. The program is applied individually, using mainly paper and pencil tasks and is based on cognitive strategy instruction. Ann Delahunty & Morice Rodney (1993) developed the first version of the program, the Frontal/Executive program, based on the specific process model. The tasks are designed to directly activate the frontal and prefrontal neural systems of the patient. The program consists of three modules: cognitive flexibility, working memory and planning (Delahunty et al. 1993, 2002).

The "Cognitive Shift Module" aims to address flexibility in thinking and information-set maintenance both of which presumably require the capacity to effectively engage and disengage activated neural network processing. It consist of a package of 6 to 8 training sessions of one hour targeting cognitive inflexibility and attention difficulties. Tasks are designed to provide some practice in exercises that help patients to get used to switching from one task to another and being able to keep in mind the information relevant to each task 'set'. It is practiced with visual, conceptual and motor information (Table 4). To ensure maintenance and the switch to the appropriate 'set' for each task, the therapist tries to use verbal instructions as a cue. Rather than performing the tasks themselves, patients should practice the connection between thought and behaviour. The therapist's task is to force the patient to pay attention to all stimuli, to ask the patient to identify what the current 'set' is and to show the patient whether their performance speed is appropriate. Finally, the therapist should promote open and covert verbal mediation of the task and not allow the patient to hesitate about what 'set' has to be used.

AREA	TARGET	INTERVENTION TECHNIQUE
Visual-motor training	Psychomotor coordination	Line bisection Cancelation tasks
Perceptual Flexibility	Alternative perceptions	Figure/Ground pictures, overlapping figures
Conceptual Flexibility	Alternative concepts	Card sorting, number shift, visual illusions, Stroop exercises
Psychomotor training	Speed Accuracy	Finger tap, hand flip, palm lifting.

Table 4. Components of the 'Cognitive shift' module.

The "Working Memory Module" aims to target the executive processes central to memory control, and has patients work with as many as two to five information sets at a time. It focuses on variables such as attention, sequencing, working simultaneously with multiple tasks, and delayed verbal and visual memory information. Working memory is defined as the ability to maintain or manipulate different sets of data. In schizophrenia, poor memorization is interpreted as a consequence of executive impairment rather than primary memory impairment per se. Thus, improving executive functions might be an important factor in enhancement of memory functioning. The module consists of two parts: A and B. Both consist of eight sessions of one hour and are designed to be used over several weeks. Part A introduces a series of working memory tasks ranging from one to four information sets. Part B provides additional exercises to Part A tasks with special emphasis on sequencing and dual tasks.

Finally, the primary target of the "Planning Module" is self-ordered, goal-oriented, set/schema formation and manipulation, that is, the application of the practiced processes, such as Working Memory, to tasks requiring planning. The goal of the tasks is to improve cognitive functioning by using active cognitive strategies including active coding, sequencing and chunking, and using internal and external verbal mediation in multitasking performance. The Planning Module also includes two parts: A and B. The first is a package of twelve sessions of one hour and part B involves about eight training sessions. Both modules provide practical exercises that facilitate the formation and manipulation of sets of information or goal-oriented schemes, with special emphasis on generating cognitive strategies and self-control. We work on control processes relating to the skills of attention, sequencing, organizing information, practical reasoning, formation of sub-objectives, and self-monitoring. Part B of the Planning Module provides more complex tasks requiring the application of effective executive skills. All tasks set out in Part B are designed to involve abstraction with more complex and complementary material. Finally, some everyday tasks like using a recipe or reading a map are used as complementary exercises.

The theoretical formulation of cognitive remediation therapy by Til Wykes and Clare Reeder (2005) also represents a major overhaul of the Frontal/Executive program. Although it uses the same treatment modules, it requires that the therapist proceed in a new way. The most important innovations are the emphasis on meta-cognition, and the use of techniques such as errorless learning and scaffolding. Scaffolding is a learning technique in which the therapist tries to teach the patient to solve problems taking their cognitive limitations into account. This involves an instructor extending a learner's ability by providing support in those aspects of a task which the learner cannot accomplish, while removing assistance in those areas where competence has been achieved. Exercises become an opportunity to practice cognitive strategies and also to learn new ones. All this learning is done through an errorless learning approach using tasks of progressive complexity and with the problem being set, as far as possible, at the subject's own pace. Subsequently, further practice is necessary to achieve the over-learning of the new cognitive strategies. The same procedure applied throughout the modules will be used to solve everyday problems of working memory, planning and, to some degree, cognitive flexibility. All in all, the treatment guidelines proposed by Wykes (2008) are based on the following principles:

1. Initial assessment
2. Identification of personal goals

3. Personal therapeutic relationship to promote self-esteem
4. Tailoring of sessions
5. Reflective learning (metacognition)
6. Use of scaffolding
7. Using errorless learning
8. Development of cognitive strategies
9. Generalization to everyday life

This program has been tested in controlled studies and has shown positive effects on cognition and on some aspects of social functioning (Wykes et al. 1999, 2007; Penadés 2006).

4.4 Studies of efficacy

The first review of cognitive remediation was performed by Kurtz et al. (2001). Because of its thoroughness and the fact that it was the first review that used meta-analytic methodology, it can be considered as a pioneering study even though, in this analysis, the authors mixed results from 'laboratory' and clinical studies. The review was conducted on three distinct cognitive domains according to the target of the neurocognitive intervention: executive function, attention and memory. Starting with executive function, a fairly statistically significant (effect size = 0.96) effect was found. Various intervention techniques produced a reduction in neurocognitive deficits such as committing perseverant errors. Furthermore, the interventions facilitate cognitive flexibility and improve patients' categorization ability. This effect remained similar in other studies despite the differences in intervention strategies. Although the meta-analysis confirmed these positive findings, the effect size obtained in clinical settings was always somewhat lower than in research conditions. Additionally, the meta-analysis showed that both reinforcement learning and teaching cognitive strategies were effective in improving performance on attention tests. Results regarding the method of repeated practice were contradictory, so their role in improving performance on attention tasks is unclear. Finally, the studies focusing on memory impairments showed that cognitive remediation is capable of enhancing memory function in a clear and consistent way, especially when the intervention is based on the teaching of coding strategies. In summary, the Kurtz study was the first to establish that cognitive intervention can produce lasting and valuable improvements in neurocognition in schizophrenia patients.

The second meta-analysis to be published was conducted by Krabbendam and German (2003). It differed considerably from the previous one in that it was the first meta-analysis performed only with controlled trials using standardized intervention protocols, comprehensive neurocognitive assessment batteries, real patients and healthy controls. The authors conducted a systematic review and chose 12 of 19 controlled studies. The main result of the analysis was that cognitive remediation was effective and produced a result considered to be a medium effect (effect size = 0.45). This finding is more or less the same as that obtained in the other review. Again, effect size was somewhat smaller in studies performed in clinical settings than in laboratory studies. Improvements were described in the majority of cognitive domains such as attention, learning and memory, verbal fluency, abstraction ability, and executive functions. On the other hand, the results were higher for programs using learning strategies than the programs using repeated practice only, although this finding did not reach statistical significance. With the publication of this study, new evidence for the efficacy neurocognitive rehabilitation was added. Specifically that neurocognitive improvement can also be obtained in clinical settings and is detectable not only in the laboratory but also in clinical neuropsychological testing. However, it still left the open question of the relevance of this improvement to daily functioning and the durability of the improvements achieved.

Almost simultaneously, Twamley et al. (2003) published another important study. These authors conducted a systematic review and decided to include only protocol-controlled studies, involving formalized intervention protocols and preferably studies carried out in clinical settings. They added another important inclusion criterion; the studies should to be randomized and assessment of the outcomes should be performed in masked conditions. Thus, it became the first meta-analysis of cognitive rehabilitation in schizophrenia with all the features of evidence-based medicine. A systematic search was conducted using these criteria with only 17 studies being selected among all studies published. In addition to efficacy on neurocognition, they compared other interesting aspects such as the type of intervention (repeated practice versus learning strategies) or whether the intervention was assisted by computer or only with paper and pencil tasks. The authors found that different types of rehabilitation were effective in improving cognitive performance and they were able to improve not only cognitive functioning but also some of the negative symptoms and daily functioning of patients. On the other hand, the programs based on computer tasks did not add better results to the use of paper and pencil tasks. However, remediation programs based on teaching strategies were more efficacious that those based only on repeated practice. As such, this meta-analysis added support to the reported efficacy of cognitive remediation programs in patients with schizophrenia, and this time the analysis was done with high-quality studies. Unfortunately, the question of whether the improvement following cognitive remediation was clinically or functionally relevant to the patient still remained an open question.

The most recent meta-analytic study was conducted by Susan McGurk et al. (2007), adding important secondary analysis to the more general analysis. It included only randomized and controlled trials, and the authors monitored neurocognition outcomes as well as clinical symptoms and psychosocial functioning. In addition, questions concerning the characteristics of rehabilitation programs were also analyzed, such as the required number of hours of intervention, the usefulness of cognitive rehabilitation programs with broader psychosocial intervention, and the importance of the patients' demographic characteristics. Other technical issues, such as the kind of control group (active or passive), were also analyzed. A total of 26 controlled studies were selected, including 1,151 patients with a diagnosis of schizophrenia. The authors underline the need for a new meta-analytic study stating that apart from the inclusion of new studies published since the last meta-analysis, previous reviews paid little attention to the effects of neurocognitive rehabilitation on psychosocial functioning.

The study confirms that cognitive remediation is effective in improving cognitive impairments in schizophrenic patients, obtaining a robust effect size (0.51), which can be considered a medium effect. This is consistent with previous studies; additionally it concluded that cognitive remediation produced an improvement in social functioning. Although the effect size was a somewhat smaller change (0.36), it can be still considered significant and medium in size. Finally, a positive effect on symptoms was also found, suggesting that there is a reduction in symptoms after rehabilitation, although the effect size is now considered only small (0.28). Thus, the study provided the first meta-analytic evidence for the impact of cognitive remediation in domains other than neurocognition. Improvements in various factors such as social functioning, quality of life, and personal autonomy were the main results. Moreover, an intuitive but previously undemonstrated hypothesis was confirmed. By adding cognitive remediation therapy to psychosocial rehabilitation, functional outcomes improved significantly. For instance, by adding cognitive remediation to vocational rehabilitation work, performance was improved and a higher level of work performance and longer-lasting jobs were generally achieved. By and large, cognitive remediation impacts on functioning only when the intervention is part of a broader psychosocial rehabilitation program. In other words, the effects of cognitive remediation therapy are higher (0.47) when acting as a part of a broader psychosocial rehabilitation than when applying cognitive remediation therapy as an isolated intervention (0.05). On the other hand, other studies have shown that cognitive remediation is clearly superior to other interventions such as occupational therapy, vocational rehabilitation programs, leisure groups, supportive therapy, watching videos, and treatment as usual. More specifically, cognitive remediation programs were more efficacious (0.62) when based on cognitive learning strategies (coaching strategy) than when the programs were based on progressive exercises or repeated practice (0.24). Learning strategies are usually based on the learning of memory strategies and cognitive abilities such as solving problems. Finally, it also was noted the improvements were shown to be maintained over periods ranging from six months to two years.

To sum up, taking into account all the current scientific evidence, we may conclude that cognitive remediation therapy is an effective treatment tool for psychiatric rehabilitation. It has been established that neurocognitive impairments can be ameliorated and some improvement in social functioning can also be expected. To achieve these results it is necessary that cognitive remediation therapy is based on the teaching of cognitive strategies and also involves some cognitive practice. Cognitive remediation therapy needs to be carried out in the context of broader psychosocial rehabilitation involving the learning of other communication, social, and self-control skills.

5. The Neuro-cognitive-behavioural approach

The majority of empirical findings, including the meta-analysis, challenge the assumption that simply improving cognitive functioning in schizophrenia will spontaneously lead to better psychosocial outcomes. Moreover, the results of previous studies suggest that cognitive remediation is probably the best option to optimize the response of some patients to psychiatric rehabilitation programs. So CRT is not likely to be implemented as a stand-alone therapy but as a part of a broader psychosocial rehabilitation program. Unfortunately, little is known about how to integrate the different rehabilitation tools in a broader rehabilitation program. Furthermore, even though these interventions show good efficacy in increasing the chances of functional improvement, only few specialized centres offer these interventions. Regrettably, they are neither standardized nor available in routine care in the majority of clinical settings.

Taking into account the published data, an evidence-based guideline for delivering cognitive remediation with other psychological treatments is presented in Figure 1. This guideline is based on the principals of the neuro-cognitive-behavioural approach established elsewhere by Penadés & Gastó (2010):

- It is an empirical approach that incorporates any sort of methodologies, learning techniques, rehabilitation programs, software or paper and pencil tasks provided that their efficacy has previously been demonstrated in controlled studies

- Rehabilitation treatment should focus on improving neurocognition but the main target is to ameliorate associated psychosocial disability
- Rehabilitation treatment must be customized for each patient and should focus on those targets considered to be important by the patient
- Rehabilitation targets should be agreed with the patient based on their capabilities, their needs and their current social environment
- This approach is called "neuro-cognitive-behavioural" since it proposes comprehensive treatment of neurocognitive aspects but does not overlook emotional, functional and psychological ones

Thus, in order to implement integrated psychosocial rehabilitation programs including CRT and evidence-based psychological therapies a flowchart has been proposed (Figure 1).

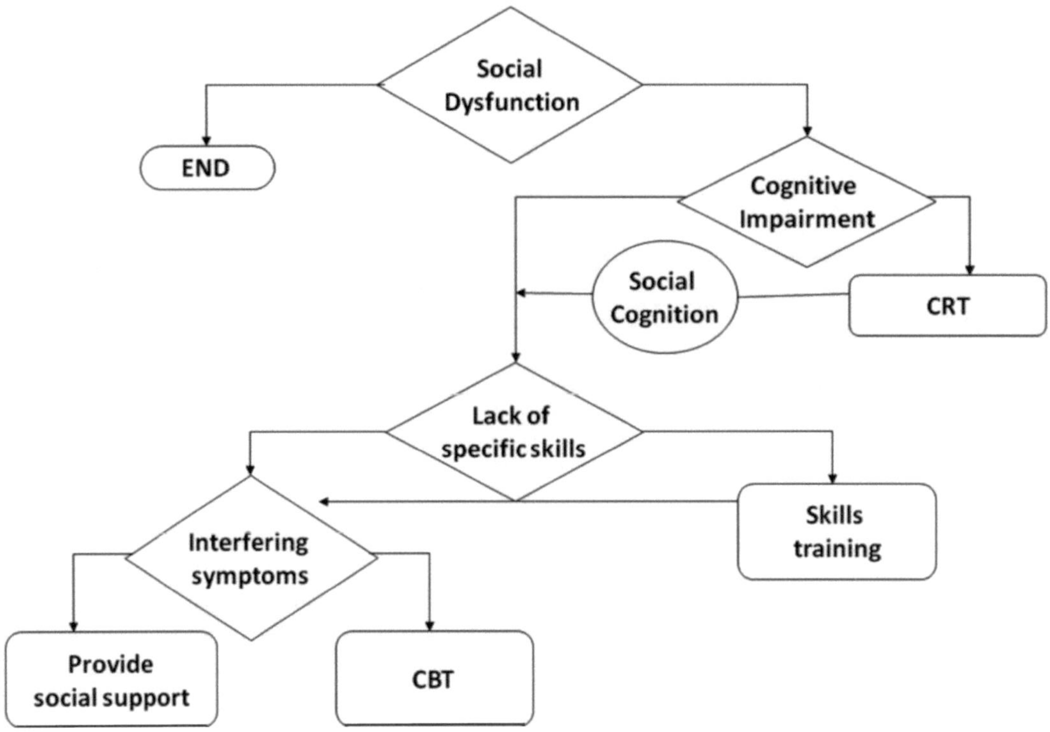

Fig. 1. Flowchart for the Neuro-cognitive-behavioural approach.

6. Improving outcomes and promoting recovery with CRT

As has been suggested before, we have some evidence that improved cognitive function can lead to improved social functioning in the context of psychological interventions. However, another concern is the identification of the cognitive domains that need to be targeted to improve functioning. In a pioneering study, Spaulding et al. (1999) investigated Integrated Psychological Therapy (IPT) (Brenner et al., 1994) and found some improvements in attention, memory, and executive function as well as improvements in social competence. However, as IPT is a multimodal program with cognitive-oriented modules and psychosocial-oriented modules, the exact role of cognitive change in overall functional improvement was not clear. In order to clarify the specific impact of cognitive change on social functioning, a controlled trial was designed (Penadés et al., 2003) using only the cognitive modules (cognitive differentiation and social perception). In this trial, memory, executive functions and social functioning showed improvement. Interestingly, changes in neurocognition were associated with changes in functional outcome, particularly in personal autonomy and general functioning.

More specifically, a number of Cognitive Remediation Therapy (CRT) studies have shown that neurocognitive improvements are associated with improvement in functioning (McGurk et al., 2007). In one of the first randomized, controlled trials comparing CRT with a control therapy, Wykes et al. (1999) found differential improvements in cognitive flexibility and memory in favour of the CRT group. When these cognitive changes reached a certain threshold, a reduction in social problems was also apparent. Furthermore, other randomized, controlled trials with CRT have shown various improvements in functioning ranging from improvements in obtaining and keeping competitive jobs (McGurk et al., 2005; Vauth et al., 2005), to the quality of, and satisfaction with, interpersonal relationships (Hogarty et al., 2004; Penadés et al., 2006) and the ability to solve interpersonal problems (Spaulding et al., 1999). These findings reinforce the assumption that neurocognition and functioning are strongly related and that CRT is useful in improving functioning.

The impact of CRT on functioning is important because the primary rationale for cognitive remediation in schizophrenia is to improve psychosocial functioning (Wykes and Reeder, 2005). Surprisingly, the majority of clinical studies of CRT did not test this hypothesis until recently and focused primarily on cognitive performance (McGurk et al., 2007). Studies have rarely investigated specific treatment mechanisms or the particular cognitive targets that are related to social improvements. Obviously, an understanding of the links between cognitive change and functional improvement is crucial in identifying appropriate cognitive targets for treatment leading to functional improvement.

In two studies, Reeder et al. (2004) published some surprising results. Cognitive functions which usually show significant cross-sectional associations with social functioning are not the same as those associated with improvement in functioning in the context of CRT. In the first study, it was found that while the "response inhibition speed" factor was associated with social functioning at baseline, change in a different factor predicted social functioning change following Cognitive Remediation Therapy (CRT). In the second study (Reeder et al., 2006), a relationship at baseline was found between social functioning and various cognitive domains such as verbal working memory, response inhibition, verbal long-term memory and visual-spatial long-term memory, but not schema generation. Surprisingly, it was the improvement in schema generation which predicted improved social functioning.

From the two studies, it can be concluded that cross-sectional associations between cognitive functions and social functioning may not be an appropriate approach for selecting cognitive targets for intervention. Even though selecting the cognitive targets of CRT on the basis of cognitive skills that appear to predict functional outcome in schizophrenia sounds logical, it could be misleading. Thus, while it has been generally assumed that improved cognition will lead to improved functional outcome, the nature of this putative link is far from clear.

Penadés et al. (2010) conducted research to investigate the neurocognitive changes occurring in the context of CRT and tried to identify which of those changes led to improvements in daily functioning. This study used data collected as part of a randomized, controlled trial investigating a CRT program in a partner study (Penadés et al., 2006). The trial recruited 52 schizophrenia patients between the ages of 27 and 42 who had been in contact with psychiatric services for at least 10 years; composing a truly chronic schizophrenia sample with predominant negative symptoms and cognitive impairments. Of these participants, 40 were randomized to receive either CRT or control psychological treatment (Cognitive Behavioral Therapy; CBT) where neurocognition was not targeted. CRT was based on the Frontal/Executive program (Delahunty and Morice, 1993). At baseline, daily functioning was significantly associated with verbal memory. Surprisingly, improvement in executive function, but not in verbal memory, predicted improved daily functioning among those with chronic schizophrenia who had current negative symptoms and evidenced neuropsychological impairments. Notwithstanding, the statistical mediation model found that social improvement caused by executive changes is expressed indirectly through improvement in verbal memory.

The direct model, as the name suggests, represents the prediction of social improvement from the change in executive function directly. The mediated model indicates that social improvement caused by executive changes is expressed indirectly through improvement in verbal memory. All variables were correlated and reached statistical significance ($\alpha > 0.05$), as can be seen in Fig. 2. None of the executive other cognitive measures, such as change in psychomotor speed (t=0.846, P=0.405), change in nonverbal memory (t=0.934, P=0.358), or change in working memory (t=1.402, P=0.172) add significant explanatory power to the effect of executive change in the social improvement function equation.

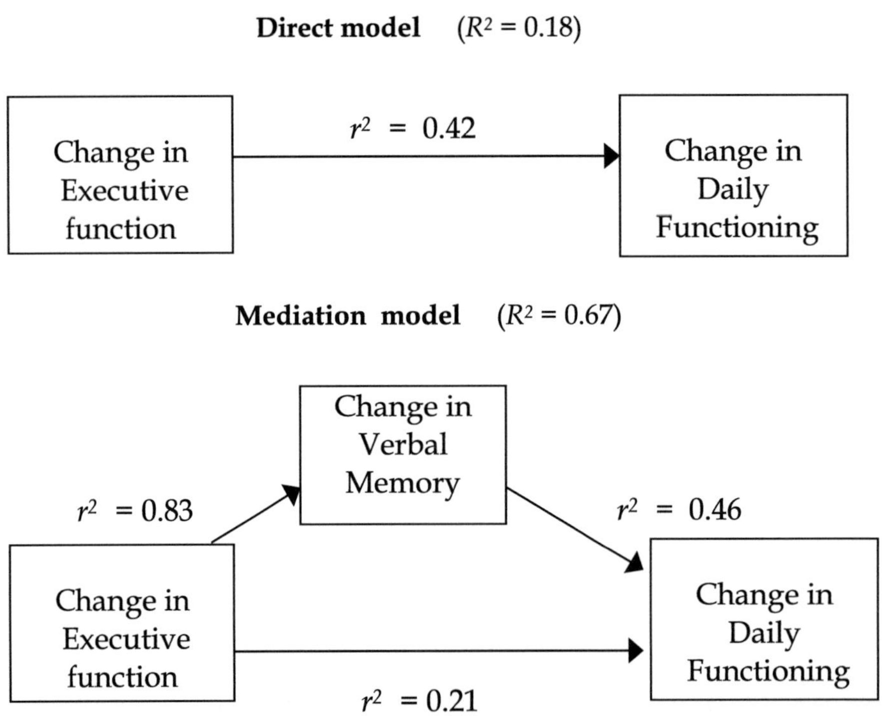

Fig. 2. Diagrams of direct and mediated models of change in daily functioning after the CRT intervention.

Thus, it was found that improvements in cognitive functions that were not significantly associated with daily functioning at baseline led to improved daily functioning. These results confirm that there is no evidence for a simple direct relationship between cognition and the different aspects of social functioning. Consequently, even if people have impairments in multiple cognitive domains, executive functioning still needs to be the intervention target. Data are consistent with findings from previous studies (Reeder et al., 2004, 2006) where it is concluded that baseline correlations may not therefore provide basic targets for intervention and may fail to highlight potential targets. In these studies, where improvements in a number of aspects of executive functioning are present, such as schema generation or response inhibition, CRT leads to improvements in social functioning regardless of baseline cognitive associations. Furthermore, it is suggested that verbal memory changes are associated with social improvements when they mediate the executive improvements. Not surprisingly, memory impairment in long-term schizophrenia can be considered as a consequence of executive impairment and not necessarily more severe cognitive impairment (Bryson et al., 2001).

7. Conclusion

Links between neurocognition and functioning have encouraged efforts to develop new pharmacological agents and novel psychological interventions targeting these variables directly. These interventions rely on the assumption that changes in neurocognition will simply improve life skills in patients with schizophrenia. This assumption is strengthened by the results of numerous studies showing that neurocognitive impairments can produce impaired social functioning. Many of these studies even suggest that neurocognitive deficits, particularly verbal memory and executive functions, are more closely linked to functional outcome than psychiatric symptoms.

However, while the role of impaired cognition in accounting for functional outcome in schizophrenia is generally established, the relationship between cognitive and functional change in the context of treatments is far from clear. In a recent study we tried to identify which cognitive changes lead to improvements in daily functioning among persons with chronic schizophrenia who had current negative symptoms and evidenced neuropsychological impairments. Cognitive Remediation Therapy (CRT) had been compared with a control therapy, involving similar length of therapist contact but different targets. At the end of treatment, CRT conferred a benefit to people with schizophrenia in cognition and functioning. Subsequently, analyses of covariance (ANCOVA) were conducted with baseline and cognitive change scores as covariates to test whether cognitive change predicted change in functioning. Additionally, statistical tests to establish the mediation path with significant variables were performed.

At baseline, daily functioning was significantly associated with verbal memory. Surprisingly, improvement in executive function, but not in verbal memory, predicted improved daily functioning among persons with chronic schizophrenia who had current negative symptoms and evidenced neuropsychological impairments. Notwithstanding, the statistical mediation model found that social improvement caused by executive changes is expressed indirectly through improvement in verbal memory. Thus, we have found that improvements in cognitive functions that were not significantly associated with daily functioning at baseline led to improved daily functioning. These results confirm that there is no evidence for a simple direct relationship between cognition and the different aspects of social functioning. Consequently, in order to improve daily functioning through CRT it is crucial to target executive function even if persons have more severe impairments in other cognitive domains. Additionally, it is important to remark that in order to achieve generalization of the CRT effects to daily functioning it is necessary to include CRT in broader programs in conjunction with other psychosocial interventions.

8. References

Andreasen, N.C. (1997). Linking Mind and Brain in the Study of Mental Illnesses: A project for a Scientific Psychopathology. *Science*. 275: 1586-1593.

American Psychiatric Association. *Diagnostic and statistical manual of mental disorders: DSM-IV*. Washington, DC: American Psychiatric Publishing, Inc.; 2000

Barch DM. (2005). The Cognitive Neuroscience of Schizophrenia. *Annual Review of Clinical Psychology*, 1: 321-353.

Bell MD, Bryson G, Greig T, Corcoran C, Wexler RE (2001) Neurocognitive enhancement therapy with work therapy. *Archives General of Psychiatry*. 58:763–768

Ben-Yishay, Y. (1980) *Working approaches to remediation of cognitive deficits in brain damaged persons: Rehabilitation monograph nº 61*. New York, University Medical Center.

Bracy, O.L. (1987) *Cognitive Rehabilitation Programs*. Indianapolis: Psychological Software Services Inc.

Brenner HD, Hodel B, Roder V, Corrigan P. (1992) Treatment of Cognitive Dysfunctions and Behavioral Deficits in Schizophrenia. *Schizophrenia Bulletin*, 18: 21-26.

Brenner, H.D., Roder, V., Hodel, B., Kienzle, N., Reed, D., Liberman, R. (1994). *Integrated Psychological Therapy for Schizophrenic Patients*. Hogrefe & Huber, Toronto, Canada.

Bryson, G., Whelahan, H.A., Bell, M. (2001). Memory and executive function impairments in deficit syndrome schizophrenia. *Psychiatry Research*, 10, 29–37.

Delahunty, A., Morice, R., (1993). *The Frontal Executive Program. A Neurocognitive Rehabilitation Program for Schizophrenia, Revised Edition*. New South Wales Department of Health, Albury, NSW, Australia.

Delahunty, A., Reeder, C., Wykes, T., Morice, R., Newton E. (2002). *Revised Cognitive Remediation Therapy Manual*. London: Institute of Psychiatry.

Green MF. (1996). What are the functional consequences of neurocognitive deficits in schizophrenia? *American Journal of Psychiatry*, 153:321-330.

Heinrichs RW, Zakzanis KK. (1998). Neurocognitive deficit in schizophrenia: a quantitative review of the evidence. *Neuropsychology*, 426-445

Hogarty, G.E., Flesher, S. (1999 a) A developmental theory for a cognitive enhancement therapy of schizophrenia. *Schizophrenia Bulletin* 25:677–692.

Hogarty, G.E., Flesher, S. (1999 b) Practice principles of cognitive enhancement therapy. *Schizophrenia Bulletin*. 25:693–708.

Hogarty, G.E., Flesher, S., Ulrich, R., Carter, M., Greenwald, D., Pogue-Geile, M., Kechavan, M., Cooley, S., DiBarry, A.L., Garret, A., Parepally, H., Zoretich, R. (2004). Cognitive enhancement therapy for schizophrenia. Effects of a 2-year randomized trial on cognition and behaviour. *Archives of General Psychiatry*, 61, 866–876.

Krabbendam, L., Aleman, A., (2003). Cognitive rehabilitation in schizophrenia: a quantitative analysis of controlled studies. *Psychopharmacology* 169, 376–382.

Kurtz MM, Moberg PJ, Gur RC, Gur RE (2001). Approaches to cognitive remediation of neuropsychological deficits in schizophrenia: A review and meta-analysis. *Neuropsychology Review*. 11: 197-210.

Lysaker, P.H., Bell, M.B., Beam-Goulet, J. (1995). Wisconsin Card Sorting Test and work performance in schizophrenia. *Psychiatry Research*. 56: 45-51.

McGurk, S.R., Meltzer, H.Y. (2003) The role of cognition in vocational functioning in schizophrenia. *Schizophrenia Research* 45: 175-184.

McGurk, S.R., Mueser, K.T., Pascaris, A. (2005). Cognitive training and supported employment for persons with severe mental illness: one year results from a randomized controlled trial. *Schizophrenia Bulletin*, 31, 898–909.

McGurk, S.R., Twamley, E.W., David, I., Sitzer, D.I., McHugo, G.J., Mueser, K.T. (2007). A meta-analysis of cognitive remediation in schizophrenia. *American Journal of Psychiatry*, 164, 1791–1802.

Pearlson, G.D., Petty, R.G., Ross, C.A. (1996) Schizophrenia: a disease of heteromodal association cortex. *Neuropsychopharmacology*. 14: 1-17.

Penadés, R., Boget, T., Catalán, R., Bernardo, M., Gastó, C., Salamero, M. (2003). Cognitive mechanisms, psychosocial functioning, and neurocognitive rehabilitation in schizophrenia. *Schizophrenia Research*, 63, 219–227.

Penadés, R., Catalán, R., Salamero, M., Boget, T., Puig, O., Guarch, J., Gastó, C. (2006). Cognitive remediation therapy for outpatients with chronic schizophrenia: a controlled and randomized study. *Schizophrenia Research*, 87, 323–331.

Penadés, R., Catalán, R., Puig, O., Masana, G., Pujol, N., Navarro, V., Guarch, J., Gastó, C. (2010) Executive function needs to be targeted to improve social functioning with Cognitive Remediation Therapy (CRT) in schizophrenia. *Psychiatry Research*. 177-41-45

Penadés, R., Gastó, C. (2010). *El tratamiento de rehabilitación neurocognitiva en la esquizofrenia*. Editorial Herder. Barcelona. (ISBN 978-84-254-2662-9).

Reeder, C., Newton, E., Frangou, S., Wykes, T. (2004). Which executive skills should we target to affect social functioning and symptom change? A study of a cognitive remediation therapy program. *Schizophrenia Bulletin*, 30, 87–100.

Reeder, C., Smedley, N., Butt, K., Bogner, D., Wykes, T. (2006). Cognitive predictors of social functioning improvements following cognitive remediation for schizophrenia. *Schizophrenia Bulletin*, 32, S123–131.

Roder V, Mueller DR, Mueser KT, Brenner HD. (2006) Integrated Psychological Therapy (IPT) for Schizophrenia: Is It Effective? *Schizophrenia Bulletin*. 32: 81–93.

Shenton, M.E., Dickey, C.C., Frumin, M., McCarley, R.W. (2001) A review of MRI findings in schizophrenia. *Schizophrenia Research*. 49: 1-52.

Spaulding, W.D., Reed, D., Sullivan, M., Richardson, C., Weiler, M. (1999). Effects of cognitive treatment in psychiatric rehabilitation. *Schizophrenia Bulletin*, 25, 657–676.

Twanley, E.W., Jeste, D.W., Bellack, A.S., (2003). A review of cognitive training in schizophrenia. *Schizophrenia Bulletin*. 29, 359–382.

Vauth, R., Corrigan, P.W., Clauss, M., Dietl, M., Dreher-Rudolph, M., Stieglitz, R.D., Vater, R. (2005). Cognitive strategies versus self-management skills as adjunct to vocational rehabilitation. *Schizophrenia Bulletin*, 31, 55–66.

Weinberger, D., Lipska, B. (1995). Cortical maldevelopment, antipsychotics drugs and schizophrenia: a search for common ground. *Schizophrenia Research*, 16, 87–110.

Wykes, T. (2008) Cognitive Rehabilitation. In Mueser, K.T. & Jeste, D.V. *Clinical Handbook of Schizophrenia.* New York: Guildford Press.

Wykes T, Reeder C, Corner J, Williams C, Everitt B (1999) The effects of neurocognitive remediation on executive processing in patients with schizophrenia. *Schizophrenia Bulletin.* 25:291–307

Wykes, T., van der Gaag, M. (2001). It is time to develop a new cognitive therapy for psychosis- Cognitive Remediation Therapy (CRT)? *Clinical Psychology Review.* 21: 1227-1256.

Wykes, T., & Reeder, C. (2005). *Cognitive Remediation Therapy: Theory and Practice,* Hove: Routledge.

Wykes T, Reeder C, Landau S, Everitt B, Knapp M, Patel A, Romeo R (2007) Cognitive remediation therapy in schizophrenia. Randomised controlled trial. *British Journal of Psychiatry.* 421-427.

5

Metacognitive Dysfunction in Schizophrenia

Martin L. Vargas*, Juan M. Sendra and Caridad Benavides
Department of Psychiatry, Complejo Asistencial de Segovia, Segovia
Spain

1. Introduction

1.1 Metacognition

Metacognition is the high-level cognitive function that can be defined as "any knowledge or cognitive process that refers to, monitors, or controls any aspect of cognition" [1]. This definition comes from developmental psychology based on Piaget's theories when Flavell, in the 1970's, used the term metamemory in regard to an individual's ability to manage and monitor the input, storage, search and retrieval of the contents of his own memory [2]. Nowadays two areas of cognitive science are included under the umbrella concept of metacognition: the knowledge of cognition (metarepresentation) and the cognitive control of the cognitive processes (executive function).

Metarepresentation is a higher-order representation of some kind [3]. That is, a metarepresentation is a representation of a representation or, in other words, knowing about knowledge. It includes such diverse aspects as auto-consciousness/self-awareness, Theory of Mind (ToM) and other diverse "meta" constructs as metamemory, metareasoning and meta-emotion or emotional intelligence. All these areas of metacognitive knowledge have in common the concept that thinking is directly focused on representations, rather than on the external world. Metarepresentation is a determinant for the human capacity of social cognition that, in schizophrenia, is a construct composed by five domains: ToM, social perception, social knowledge, attributional bias and emotion processing [4]. Finally, constructing the narrative of self-identity largely depends on social cognition [5]. Scholl and Lesley [6] propose that ToM relies on the function of one specific brain module. Conceived in the classical way modules are defined as an innate, encapsulated and domain-specific part of the cognitive architecture, but with the characteristic of being a 'diachronic' module with the dynamic capacity to attain its character from the environment. This ToM module is the basic cognitive function that capacitates the four other more molar metarepresentative domains of the social human brain. Although the detailed implementation of the ToM module still remains unknown, probably it implies areas of complex cerebral connectivity [7] in the core circuit for imitation provided with neurons with mirror properties: posterior inferior frontal gyrus, ventral premotor cortex, the rostral part of the inferior parietal lobule and posterior sector of the superior temporal sulcus [8]. Analyzing data from functional neuroimaging, Gallagher and Frith [9] conclude that the ability to mentalize is mediated

---

*Corresponding Author

more concretely by a circumscribed region of the anterior paracingulate cortex. This region seems to be strongly associated with a more widespread network of cerebral regions involved in social cognition including the amygdala and the orbital frontal cortex.

Cognitive control, executive function or executive control, on the other hand, is the constellation of cognitive processes closely related to the frontal lobe functioning that monitors and controls cognition. It is composed of three independent but related dimensions: shifting between mental sets or tasks (Shifting), updating and monitoring of working memory contents (Updating), and inhibition of prepotent responses (Inhibition) [10]. Executive functioning is needed for any complex cognitive demand. It is genetically determined to a high degree and closely depends on dopamine neurotransmission [11] as well as the connectivity between network nodes of frontoparietal and frontostriatal circuits [12]. But, contrary to the case of ToM, and due to its heterarchical associative nature, executive function does not meet the characteristics to be implemented in one brain module. The brain cortex is functionally structured in cognits, which can be defined as "an item of knowledge about the world, the self, or the relations between them" [13]. A cognit is made up of groups of neurons and the connections between them. As more complex cognitive demands are required, the associative cognits of higher hierarchy are activated in the perception-action cycle. Cognitive functions overlap with each other from the simpler to the more complex and human-specific at the top of the hierarchy. So, the executive control in one perception-action cycle constitutes what Fuster [13] names as the high-level cognit that is broadly distributed in associative cortical areas or what Fodor years ago refered to as the one central process which does not have a modular architecture [14].

In brief, we differentiate two components in metacognition: a) the module for ToM, which is the core of social cognition and self identity and b) executive control, which is not modular but depends on broad cortical connectivity, and acts as the mediator factor integrating ToM in the global function of cognition. Executive dysfunction [15, 16] and ToM deficits [17, 18] have been confirmed as important conditions in schizophrenia. Furthermore, they are key concepts in the development of new evidence-based psychological treatments for schizophrenia, such as, Metacognitive training (MCT) [19] or Cognitive Remediation Therapy (CRT) [20], where improvement in daily functioning was predicted by better executive functioning [21] achieved by modifying metacognitive thinking strategies. So, improved knowledge of the metacognitive disturbances in schizophrenia appears to be a promising topic with high clinical and research interest.

1.2 Metacognitive deficits in schizophrenia

At the neurotransmission level, dopamine abnormalities appear to be related to schizophrenia both in metacognitive and social cognitive disorders as well as in executive disorders. Oxytocinergic and dopaminergic signalling in the amygdala result in impaired emotional salience and consequent social cognitive disturbance [22]. Dopamine presynaptic abnormality is the "final common pathway" causing the aberrant salience that is the gateway in to the psychosis [23] and is still considered the main target in the pharmacological treatment of the disease. At a higher level of analysis, social cognitive networks, executive control networks and the speech-related resting state network, have abnormal connectivity [24]. Executive function is the most global cognitive function and its deficit in schizophrenia is well known from the early states of the disease as well as in non-affected first degree relatives [15, 16]. Moreover, executive dysfunction is closely related to the dopamine and other monoamine genetic differences that could mediate one important component of the genetic risk to the disease [11].

The impact of this deficit on the different domains of social cognition has been studied. Couture et al [25] propose that deficits in ToM could cause hostility-biased attributional style thereby leading to problems with social cognition and consequently the social functioning of the subject. This term has been partially confirmed by a path analysis study that found ToM to be a partial mediator between global neurocognition and social competence [26]. However, the hostile attributional style is only related to symptoms, ToM and social cue detection deficits being the two dimensions most closely correlated with functional outcome [27]. How much of the ToM deficit in schizophrenia is due to executive dysfunction has been a heated topic of debate, similar to what has happened in other diseases with cognitive dysfunction. For example, comparing bipolar patients to healthy controls, the worse execution of ToM tasks remains significant after controlling for executive dysfunction [28]. In another study [29], ToM problems were more closely related to attention disorders than executive dysfunction, ToM appearing as a state marker but not as a trait of the disease. So, ToM deficit seems to be dissociated from executive dysfunction in bipolar disorder. But in Parkinson's disease, the independence of ToM disorders from other cognitive dimensions is not as clear. Peron et al [30] found a significant correlation between the Stroop interference score and a subscore of the faux pas recognition test (explanation score) and argue that ToM impairments in advanced PD patients could be the consequence of general cognitive deterioration and that the dysexecutive syndrome could explain the mental state inference deficit. In a similar way, it has been proposed that ToM dysfunction schizophrenia may reflect impairments in related non-ToM abilities, such as executive functioning, rather than representing a specific ToM deficit [17]. Those models proposing that poor performance in ToM tasks in healthy and clinical populations [31] reflect executive dysfunction argue that it could be due to the difficulty to disengage from and inhibit salient information or, on the other hand, be due to problems in the manipulation of representations of hypothetical situations. The former case relates mainly to shifting and inhibition dimensions of executive functioning and can be evaluated by the Wisconsin Card Sorting Test, while the latter indicates problems with updating working memory which is evaluated by the Tower of London task. The relationship between ToM and executive function has been systematically reviewed by Pickup [32] who refers consistently to the question indicating that specifically impaired ToM in schizophrenia actually exists reflecting dysfunction of a domain-specific cognitive system, rather than only a domain-general executive impairment. The author concludes that executive function and ToM are independent in schizophrenia, leading to the independent contribution of ToM in functioning. Furthermore, ToM impairments appear to be both a trait and state deficit.

The current state of knowledge points out that ToM constitutes a brain module that can be independently affected in schizophrenia constituting a domain-specific ToM deficit. But this fact is not incompatible with the coexistence of domain-nonspecific metacognitive deficits. Social perception, social knowledge, attributional bias and emotion processing are social cognition domains that, although based on ToM, depend on other basic and executive cognitive functions that also require wide brain connectivity. Schizophrenia has been proposed to reflect the disconnection syndrome of the highest hierarchy human networks such as those implicated in social cognition and Theory of Mind (ToM) [7]. Multimodal network organization is abnormal in schizophrenia, as indicated by reduced hierarchy, the loss of frontal and the emergence of nonfrontal hubs, and increased connection distance [33]. These authors defined the anatomical networks, studying inter-regional correlations of high-resolution magnetic resonance image, revealing the usefulness of correlation techniques in the study of cortical functional networks. So, in conjunction with the domain-specific ToM deficit, other domain-nonspecific metacognitive dysfunction due to disconnection of associative cortical areas could exist, acting as a moderator variable on the effect of ToM deficits in the pathophysiology of schizophrenia. The association of dysfunction in the module for ToM jointly with executive dysfunctions due to cortical disconnection could increase the risk for clinical schizophrenia in vulnerable people. In this manner, the dopaminergic ToM dysfunction acts as the necessary cause or vulnerability trait of the disease, while the increased effect due to the coexistence of cortical disconnection leads to the effect from the trait of vulnerability to the state of clinical schizophrenia.

The objective of this review is to determine candidate domain-nonspecific metacognitive deficits in schizophrenia. We will investigate the association described in the schizophrenia literature between executive and metarepresentative dysfunctions and we will show that the domains of executive function and metarepresentation which are linked to a large size effect constitute a network that, when connectivity decreases, leads to domain-nonspecific metacognitive deficits.

2. Method

We have done a systematic review on PubMed and PsychoInfo in August, 30th 2011 introducing the following syntax. PubMed: Schizophrenia [MeSH Terms] AND (("dysexecutive"[All Fields] AND ("syndrome"[MeSH Terms] OR "syndrome"[All Fields])) OR executive [All Fields] OR frontal [All fields]) AND ("Theory of Mind" [All Fields] OR "metacognition" [All Fields] OR "metarepresentation" [All Fields] OR "social cognition" [All Fields]). PsychoInfo: Schizophrenia AND (dysexecutive OR executive OR frontal) AND ("Theory of Mind" OR metacognition OR metarepresentation OR "social cognition").

The obtained articles were reviewed by reading the abstracts. Articles were selected for full reading when the abstracts refered directly or indirectly to any association measure as correlation, regression, odds ratio or risk ratio between metarepresentation and executive function in schizophrenia. After that, the articles were definitively included if they provided the association measure. Finally, only the associations with large effect size were considered for analysis. The criteria for considering the effect size was that proposed by Cohen who accepts $r \geq 0.5$ (shared variance equal or greater than 0.25) as a large effect size [34]. These will be our proposed domain non-specific metacognitive deficits.

3. Results

Sixty-five articles were obtained from PubMed and 125 from PsycInfo. After abstract reading, 36 were fully read and 14 were definitively included in the analysis. Table 1 shows the article references and their main characteristics and results. All of them were published after 2000. Most of the works explores the relationship between ToM and executive function as secondary, not the main objective. Only Lysaker et al [35] specifically evaluated this relationship. The measuring instruments used are highly variable, especially in ToM, where there is little overlap between studies. Regarding the instruments used to assess executive function, the Wisconsin Card Sorting Test (WCST) is highlighted. It is used in half of the studies. As a relational measure the authors uses the correlation coefficient in 86% of the studies, one used analysis of covariance (ANCOVA) and one used linear regression. Most authors do not specify what type of correlation coefficient is chosen, except in three specific cases (two works with Pearson's correlation coefficient and one with Spearman's coefficient).

Reference Country	ToM measuring instruments	Executive function measuring instruments	Relation measuring Results
[42] Australia	Mind in the Eyes test -ME-	Reality-unknown (low-inhibition false belief -LOFB-) task. Reality-known (high-inhibition false belief -HIFB-) task.	Correlation ME/LOFB: .40* ME/HIFB: .38* *: p<.05
[43] United States	Bell Lysaker Emotion Recognition Test (BLERT) total score. Hinting Task total score. Bell Object Relations Inventory (BORI) Egocentricity Scale. Rapport item on the Quality of Life Scale (QLS).	Wisconsin Card Sorting Test (WCST).	Correlation BLERT/WCST: .184* Hinting/WCST: .260*** BORI/WCST: .169* QLS/WCST: .115 (ns) *:p< .05 ***:p< .001
[38] Germany	Ekman and Friesen's Pictures of Facial Affect. ToM novel series: *ToM questionnaire; ToM total score.*	Wisconsin Card Sorting Test (WCST). Behavioural Assessment of the Dysexecutive Syndrome (BADS): *Key Search Test (KST); Zoo Map Test (ZMT).*	Correlation ToM/WCST errors: -.114 (ns) ToM/WCSTpers: -.354 (ns) ToM/KST: .605** ToM/ZMT: .492* *:p< .05; **:p< .01 Correlations with ToM total score.
[44] United States	Facial Emotion Identification Test (FEIT).	Wisconsin Card Sorting Task (WCST).	Correlation FEIT/WCST: .34 (ns)
[45] Japan	Role-play test (RPT) including fifteen parameters.	Trail Making Test (TMT) A and B: *differences in score B – A.*	Spearman's correlation RPT (Recognition of goal)/TMT: -.36* RPT(Generating thought)/TMT: -.36* *: p=.01

Reference Country	**ToM measuring instruments**	**Executive function measuring instruments**	**Relation measuring Results**
[41] United States	Means-Ends Problem-Solving (MEPS). Social Cue Recognition Test (SCRT): *concrete false-positive errors (CFPE) and abstract false-positive errors (AFPE).*	Wisconsin Card Sorting Task (WCST).	Correlation MEPS/WCST: .35* SCRT(CFPE)/WCST: -.57** SCRT(AFPE)/WCST -.56** *:p< .05; **:p< .0001
[31] Australia	Picture-sequencing task: *False-belief mean position score (FBmps) (mentalising ability).*	Computerised version of the Tower of London task: *Proportion of ToL problems solves in the minimum (Min); Number of moves taken beyond the minimum (Moves); Initial planning time (Init); Subsequent planning time (Sub).*	Correlation FBmps /Min: .38 (ns) FBmps /Moves: -.25 (ns) FBmps /Init: -.15 (ns) FBmps /Sub: -.26 (ns)
[39] Australia	Picture-sequencing task (false-belief picture-sequencing score): FB-ps. Non-literal speech comprehension by computerized story comprehension task: *(metaphor hit rate): Met-hit; (irony hit rate): Iron-hit.*	Picture-sequencing task (*capture picture-sequencing score): C-ps* Computerized version of the Tower of London: *(% ToL problems solved in min. no. of moves*): *ToL%;* (*average no. moves taken on ToL task*): *ToL-mov;* (*subsequent planning time on ToL task*): *ToL-sub.*	Correlation FB-ps/ C-ps: .57** FB-ps/ ToL-mov:-.46* FB-ps/ ToL-sub: -.58** Met-hit/ToL-sub: -.44* Iron-hit/ToL-mov: -.40* Iron-hit/ToL%: -.42* *:p< .05; **:p<.01
[35] United States	Metacognition Assessment Scale (MAS): *Understanding one's own mind (UOwM); Understanding the others' mind (UOtM); Mastery (M); Total (T).*	Delis Kaplan Executive Function System (DKEFS): *Design Fluency Switching (DFS); Verbal Fluency Switching (VFS); Color Word Switching (CWS); Sorting Task (ST); Word Context (WC); Twenty Questions (TQ).*	Spearman's correlation UOwM/ST: .47** UOwM/WC: .47** UOwM/TQ: .32* UOtM/DFS: .30* UOtM/DFS: .31* M/VFS: .31* M/TQ: .32* T/VFS: .34* T/TQ: .43** *:p< .05; **:p< .01

Reference Country	ToM measuring instruments	Executive function measuring instruments	Relation measuring Results
[40] Germany	Computerized series of six picture stories (PS).	Wisconsin Card Sorting Test (WCST): *perseverative errors.* Behavioural Assessment of the Dysexecutive Syndrome (BADS): *Zoo Map Test.*	Parametric correlation PS/WCST(FP): .60** PS/BADS(FP): .35* PS/WCST(NFP): .49** PS/WCST(NFP) .487** *:p<.05; **:p<.01 FP: forensic patients; NFP: nonforensic patients.
[46] Italy	First-Order ToM Tasks (F-Or-T). Second-Order ToM Tasks (S-Or-T).	Tower of London test (TL). Phonemic verbal fluency test (PVF).	ANCOVA F-Or-T/TL: F= .46 (ns) F-Or-T/PVF: F= .35 (ns) S-Or-T/TL: F= .16 (ns) S-Or-T/PVF: F= .18 (ns)
[37] Italy	Comprehensive Affect Testing System (CATS).	Wisconsin Card Sorting Test (WCST).	Univariate linear regression analyses CATS/WCST: $\beta = .276$, $p = .04$ $\beta^* = .253$, $p^* = .048$ *: *: partial regression analyses excluding face perception.
[47] United Kingdom	Theory-of-mind (ToM) task.	Wisconsin Card Sorting Test (WCST).	Pearson's correlation ToM/WCST: -.46 p=.01
[36] Norway	Emotion perception (EP): *Visual emotion identification; Visual emotion discrimination; Auditory emotion identification; Auditory emotion discrimination.* (Z-transformed composite score based on principal components analysis is the measure of emotion perception).	Neurocognition (NC): *Psychomotor speed (Digit Symbol; SS); Semantic fluency (Animals & Boys' Names; SS); Executive control (Inhibition/Switching; SS); Verbal learning (CVLT-II; T-score).* SS: Scaled score; T-Score: Total score. (Z-transformed composite score based on principal components analysis is the measure of neurocognition).	Pearson correlation EP/NC: .67 p=.01

Table 1. Selected articles for analysis.

In connection to the results found there is great variability, generally showing positive correlations with significant results in those papers that perform multiple comparisons. Studies with negative correlations in their comparisons or no significant results are detected. Probably this high variability is conditioned by the variety of measuring instruments used by different authors, as the mention of ToM does not coincide in any author. Another factor explaining this phenomenon is probably the definition applied by different authors in the conceptualization of the term ToM and executive function, which leads to the use of different instruments as mentioned previously.

Six of the selected fourteen studies report any large effect size correlation. Three of them refer to emotion processing [36-38], two refer to ToM [39, 40] and one paper refers to social perception [41]. Studies were not detected with correlations between executive dysfunction and social knowledge or attributional bias. The results of our review show that executive dysfunction could act as a mediator or moderator variable on the clinical consequences of the domain-specific ToM deficit. In addition, emotion and social processing problems can be proposed as candidate domain-nonspecific deficits highly influenced by executive dysfunction.

3.1 Executive dysfunction influencing the effect of ToM deficits

Although ToM deficits constitute an independent and probably modular dysfunction in schizophrenia, it is not free from intermediate variables affecting its clinical manifestation. One study [40] evaluated ToM abilities using a computerized series of six picture stories depicting the cooperation of two characters, one character deceiving another, or two characters cooperating to deceive a third. It revealed that in a sample of forensic schizophrenia patients, ToM task performance inversely correlated with the amount of WCST perseverative errors ($r = -0.598$, $p < 0.001$) and with the performance on the Zoo Map Test ($r = 0.346$, $p = 0.048$), a subtest taken from the Behavioural Assessment of the Dysexecutive Syndrome (BADS). The results were similar in other samples of nonforensic schizophrenia patients. Another study testing the effect of mind-reading on the pragmatic language impairments in schizophrenia [39] observed that the performance in the mind-reading task was related to executive functioning. The task used to study mind-reading was a picture-sequencing task. Stories were presented on cards referring to four experimental story types: social-script stories testing logical reasoning about people without needing to infer mental states, mechanical stories testing physical cause-and-effect reasoning, false-belief stories testing general mind-reading, and capture stories testing inhibitory control. Executive functioning was tested using the capture picture-sequencing score to measure inhibitory control and a version of the Tower of London (ToL) task to measure planning. As a secondary result of the study, it was observed that executive dysfunction (errors in sequencing capture stories and poor ToL task performances) predicted mind-reading impairments and pragmatic comprehension deficits in schizophrenic patients. The association was $r = -0.57$ ($p<0.01$) for false-belief picture-sequencing and capture picture-sequencing, and $r = -0.58$ ($p<0.01$) for false-belief picture-sequencing and subsequent planning time on ToL task. But the effect of mind-reading on pragmatic comprehension deficits does not depend on executive dysfunction as this persists after controlling for executive functioning in a logistic regression model. So, in this case an independent ToM disorder appears causing the pragmatic language deficits in addition or independently from the executive dysfunction, but is not mediated by it. The same study concludes that executive dysfunction and, beyond that, a selective difficulty with interpreting metaphors (most likely due to abnormal semantics) were associated with negative formal thought disorders, whereas positive formal thought disorders were associated with poor mind-reading. Its different clinical manifestation supports the differentiation between executive and ToM disorders.

These two studies are examples of executive dysfunction associated with ToM deficits. Executive dysfunction could affect the impact of ToM deficits in several result variables, as symptoms or functioning do. But we should determine if executive dysfunction acts as a modulating or as a mediating factor. A modulating factor modifies the size effect of the independent variable on the dependent variable. To our knowledge, the potential role of executive dysfunction as the moderator of the effect of ToM on symptoms or functioning is still unknown. On the other hand, a mediating effect is said to be present if the mediator is related to the independent and dependent variables and, furthermore, if a previously significant relationship between the independent and the dependent variables is no longer significant, or at least greatly reduced, when the mediator is controlled. This is not the case in the study of Langdon et al [39], which shows that the effect of ToM disorders on formal thought disorders persists after controlling the executive functioning.

We can conclude that, although sufficient evidence exists leading to the acceptance of the independence of the effects of ToM deficits on several clinical and functional targets, probably in some situations executive dysfunction can play a role as a modulating factor. In other cases it will be a merely coexistent deficit, but we can exclude that executive dysfunction acts as a mediator factor between ToM deficits and its functional and clinical consequences. In any case, the best way to characterise ToM deficits in schizophrenia is considering it a domain-specific deficit.

3.2 Executive dysfunction causing emotion processing problems

The result of our review suggests emotion processing problems as the most firm candidates for a domain-nonspecific deficit, defined as a deficit not depending on any single cognitive module dysfunction, but related to problems in the interaction or connection between diverse modules. Three of the selected studies address this topic.

The first of them [38] follows the proposal of Frith [48] who hypothesized that many symptoms typical of schizophrenia may be accounted for by a specific cognitive incapacity of schizophrenic patients to accurately attribute mental states to themselves or others, leading to disorders of willed action, disorders of self-monitoring and disorders of monitoring other persons thoughts and intentions. Brüne highlights the importance of differentiating non-social versus social cognitive testing in the study of schizophrenia since the latter may distinguish between patients and nonpatients better [49]. Considering that the perception of emotional states involves a ventral brain stream (amygdala and orbitofrontal cortex) whereas a dorsal pathway (superior temporal sulcus, inferior frontal regions, medial prefrontal cortex including parts of the anterior cingulate cortex) relates to ToM, the study aims to show the amount of explained variance of the patients' actual social behavioural abnormalities which are due to emotion recognition and ToM capacities. The results reveal that schizophrenic patients differed significantly from healthy controls in the main measures of executive functioning, emotion recognition, and ToM. However, after controlling for executive functioning (as measured by perseverative errors on the WCST) and IQ, the effect disappears in happiness, fear and sadness recognition. In this case, executive functioning seems to be a mediating factor between non-social cognitive capacities and emotion perception. Furthermore, ToM and emotion recognition were not related to executive functioning in the healthy subjects of the control group while moderate associations appeared in the schizophrenic group, supporting executive functioning to be related to emotion perception and ToM only in the disease condition. The author concludes that the slowing of patient performance of ToM tasks is partly associated with their impaired understanding of the social interaction depicted in the stories, and with executive functioning. To determine the contribution of ToM and executive performance in the assignation to the schizophrenia group, a logistical regression analysis (backward-step) was done. Although ToM performance remained in the equation as the most powerful predictor of the odds of being in the group of patients, the number of perseverative errors in the computerized WCST also remained significant, but did not correlate with ToM performance in the patient group. The results of this study suggest independent contributions of ToM and executive functioning and support the differentiation we make between domain-specific and domain-nonspecific dysfunctions.

A second study [36] addressed specifically social cognition and learning potential as mediating variables between neurocognition and functional outcome in schizophrenia and confirmed that emotion perception has a mediating role in the association between neurocognition and social problem-solving. The authors propose that the mediating role that social cognition plays between neurocognition and functioning could be due to the recognition of emotional expressions in other people, probably depending on basic neurocognitive abilities such as working memory, visual scanning, and speech and face perception. To measure non-social cognition, a composite battery based on MATRICS was used, including Digit Symbol, Semantic Fluency, Inhibition/Switching and California Verbal Learning Test-II, Total List A learning. Emotion perception was assessed using the Face/Voice Emotion Identification and Discrimination Test that requires the identification of emotions from six alternatives in facial pictures and tape-recorded sentences. As functional outcome variable, a social problem-solving test was used. Emotion perception confirmed its mediating role in this study through its significant relation to both the independent (neurocognition: $r=.67$, $p<.001$) and the dependent variable (social problem solving, $r=.50$, $p< .001$) in conjunction with the elimination of the effect of neurocognition on social problem-solving when controlling for emotion perception in a regression analysis. The results are in line with other studies which have found that facial affect recognition is a partial mediator between neurocognition and social functioning (quality of life) in psychosis [50] or that social perception mediates between neurocognition and interpersonal role-playing skills [51].

The third study related to emotion processing which our review detected is by Rocca et al [37]. Its aim was to study the role of facial identity recognition in the context of cognitive functions and symptoms considering that facial emotion recognition deficits may be part of a cognitive impairment in the domains of attention and executive functions. The executive assessment was done with the Stroop Test, the Trail Making Test and the Wisconsin Card Sorting Test (WCST). Facial emotion processing assessment used the Comprehensive Affect Testing System (CATS). The results of the study support the presence of a generalized deficit where both facial recognition and facial emotion recognition were affected in schizophrenia. Using linear regression analysis the authors conclude that executive dysfunction may explain a proportion of the variance in emotion recognition in conjunction with attention, face perception and verbal memory-learning. Executive functions explained 7% of the variance in emotion perception scores. In this case, the coincidence of diverse basic cognitive capacities is the cause of emotion perception deficits that we categorize as domain non-specific metacognitive deficits.

Emotion processing deficits appears to be the best candidate in a domain non-specific metacognitive deficit, which in part is due to executive dysfunction. Executive dysfunction has been viewed to act both as a causal factor in addition to other, as well as being a mediating factor between non-social cognition and emotion perception.

3.3 Executive dysfunction causing social processing problems

One study has been found with a relevant association between social cognition and executive functioning [41]. It studied the relationships between various domains of neurocognition and two forms of social cognition (social cue recognition and social problem solving) in patients with schizophrenia spectrum disorders. The study was based on the hypothesis that executive function is related to abstract cue recognition and social problem solving because both forms of social cognition require the ability to think in an abstract and flexible manner about diverse situations. After controlling for symptomatology, perseverative errors in the WCST accounted for 22% of the variance in a task of social cue recognition and 11% in a task of social problem-solving. The authors conclude that deviations in neurocognition may affect the ability of persons to recognize the intentions of others in common social situations, specifically when they are communicated in a more implicit manner. The social cue recognition deficits can occur via executive dysfunction, or but by other means, such as attention or memory deficits.

Social processing, similar to emotion processing, is not a simple or modular cognitive process but a complex capacity. Executive dysfunction probably affects social processing, acting as a causal or mediating factor but there is still little evidence to prove that. So, we accept deficits in social processing as a putative non-specific metacognitive deficit in schizophrenia.

3.4 Future research

ToM is a modular cognitive capacity relatively independent from its interrelation with other capacities which may be primarily altered in schizophrenia, specifically in those cases with predominance of autistic symptoms. The analysis of potential common endophenotypes shared by autism and a subgroup of schizophrenic patients appears to be an exciting area of research into metacognition and psychosis.

However, probably the most interesting area for further research is that of non-specific metacognitive disorders. First of all, a more detailed knowledge of the social cognitive domains that can be mediated or caused by executive dysfunction is necessary. Considering ToM to be the most nuclear social cognitive domain closely related to its specific module, emotion processing and social perception appear to be complex domains where the impact of connectivity pathology on executive functioning may be an important target for new studies. As executive functioning highly depends on dopaminergic neurotransmission and cortical connectivity [52], it could be found to be an important common pathway in the pathophysiology of the disease linking dopamine or glial disorders [53] to metarepresentative symptoms via executive dysfunction.

Social knowledge and attributional bias did not appear as candidates to be related to executive dysfunction or to metarepresentation disorders. We consider them to be basically related to episodic and semantic memory, being the final product of experience. Both are close to the thinking style of the patient, with his or her cognitive traits, but do not relate to the neurocognitive substrata of the disease.

Social cognition is a confirmed mediator between neurocognition and functioning. Metarepresentation is the key concept used to study social cognition and executive functioning. We propose to take into account the different nature of each of the five dimensions of social cognition in schizophrenia. ToM would be the basic cognitive module affected, which is an endophenotype and hence its dysfunction remains stable over time with little or no modification due to treatment. Executive dysfunction is due to dopamine or connectivity alterations and may act as a modulating or mediating factor when ToM disorders are the primary cause of the metacognitive disorder. Executive dysfunction could also be a causing factor independent from ToM. Emotion processing and social perception are domains more closely affected by executive dysfunction and probably both of them behave like state markers. Thus, they can be expected to fluctuate with clinical episodes and pharmacological treatments. Finally, social knowledge and attributional bias, as they relate to semantic knowledge and cognitive schemas, could be good candidates for improvement through psychotherapy. These speculations could serve as a guide for further research.

4. Conclusion

Metacognitive disorders in schizophrenia are central to the pathophysiology and psychopathology of the disease. ToM disorders are domain-specific and are related to a particular cognitive module. This chapter systematically reviews the literature on metarepresentation and executive dysfunction in schizophrenia to determine candidate domain-nonspecific metacognitive deficits. Emotion processing problems have been detected to be the best candidate. Executive dysfunction seems to be a mediating or causing factor that causes emotion processing problems which consequently lead to functioning deficits or symptom exacerbation. Social processing could be another non-specific metacognitive disorder but less evidence to sustain this term exists.

Social cognition acts as a mediator between non-social cognition and functioning. But social cognition itself is a heterogeneous construct that must be studied taking into account metacognition, basic cognition and personality traits. An in-depth analysis of this topic could contribute to a better understanding of this new and exciting area of research in schizophrenia. We propose to consider ToM the nuclear metacognitive dimension. Emotion and social perception are domains based on ToM but highly dependant on connectivity and on executive functioning. And finally, attributional bias and social knowledge could depend on personality traits more than on metacognition.

5. References

[1] Moses, L.J. and J.A. Baird, Metacognition., in The MIT Encyclopedia of the Cognitive Sciences, R.A. Wilson and F. Keil, Editors. 1999, MIT Press: Cambridge, MA. p. 533–535.

[2] Flavell, J., Metacognition and cognitive monitoring; A new area of cognitive-developmental inquiry. American Psychologist, 1979. 34: p. 906-911.

[3] Dennett, D.C., Making tools for thinking, in Metarepresentations: A Multidisciplinary Perspective, D. Sperber, Editor. 2000, Oxford University Press: New York.

[4] Green, M.F., et al., Social cognition in schizophrenia: an NIMH workshop on definitions, assessment, and research opportunities. Schizophr Bull, 2008. 34(6): p. 1211-20.

[5] Kircher, T. and A. David, eds. The Self in Neuroscience and Psychiatry. 2003, Cambridge University Press: Cambridge.

[6] Scholl, B. and A. Leslie, Modularity, Development and 'Theory of Mind'. Mind & Language, 1999. 14(1): p. 131-53.

[7] Burns, J.K., An evolutionary theory of schizophrenia: cortical connectivity, metarepresentation, and the social brain. Behav Brain Sci, 2004. 27(6): p. 831-55; discussion 855-85.

[8] Bermúdez, J., Cognitive Science. An introduction to the Science of the Mind. 2010, Cambridge: Cambridge University Press.

[9] Gallagher, H.L. and C.D. Frith, Functional imaging of 'theory of mind'. Trends Cogn Sci, 2003. 7(2): p. 77-83.

[10] Miyake, A., et al., The unity and diversity of executive functions and their contributions to complex "Frontal Lobe" tasks: a latent variable analysis. Cogn Psychol, 2000. 41(1): p. 49-100.

[11] Barnes, J.J., et al., The molecular genetics of executive function: role of monoamine system genes. Biol Psychiatry, 2011. 69(12): p. e127-43.

[12] Tau, G.Z. and B.S. Peterson, Normal development of brain circuits. Neuropsychopharmacology, 2010. 35(1): p. 147-68.

[13] Fuster, J., Cortex and Mind. Unifying Cognition. 2005, New York: Oxford University Press.

[14] Fodor, J.A., The Modularity of Mind. 1983, Cambridge, MA: MIT Press.

[15] Freedman, D. and A.S. Brown, The developmental course of executive functioning in schizophrenia. Int J Dev Neurosci, 2011. 29(3): p. 237-43.

[16] Eisenberg, D.P. and K.F. Berman, Executive function, neural circuitry, and genetic mechanisms in schizophrenia. Neuropsychopharmacology, 2010. 35(1): p. 258-77.

[17] Bora, E., M. Yucel, and C. Pantelis, Theory of mind impairment: a distinct trait-marker for schizophrenia spectrum disorders and bipolar disorder? Acta Psychiatr Scand, 2009. 120(4): p. 253-64.

[18] Lysaker, P.H., et al., Metacognition in schizophrenia: Correlates and stability of deficits in theory of mind and self-reflectivity. Psychiatry Res, 2010.

[19] Moritz, S., et al., Further evidence for the efficacy of a metacognitive group training in schizophrenia. Behav Res Ther, 2011. 49(3): p. 151-7.

[20] Wykes, T., et al., A meta-analysis of cognitive remediation for schizophrenia: methodology and effect sizes. Am J Psychiatry, 2011. 168(5): p. 472-85.

[21] Penades, R., et al., Executive function needs to be targeted to improve social functioning with Cognitive Remediation Therapy (CRT) in schizophrenia. Psychiatry Res, 2010. 177(1-2): p. 41-5.

[22] Rosenfeld, A.J., J.A. Lieberman, and L.F. Jarskog, Oxytocin, dopamine, and the amygdala: a neurofunctional model of social cognitive deficits in schizophrenia. Schizophr Bull, 2010. 37(5): p. 1077-87.

[23] Howes, O.D. and S. Kapur, The dopamine hypothesis of schizophrenia: version III--the final common pathway. Schizophr Bull, 2009. 35(3): p. 549-62.

[24] Wolf, N.D., et al., Dysconnectivity of multiple resting-state networks in patients with schizophrenia who have persistent auditory verbal hallucinations. J Psychiatry Neurosci, 2011. 36(6): p. 366–374.

[25] Couture, S.M., D.L. Penn, and D.L. Roberts, The functional significance of social cognition in schizophrenia: a review. Schizophr Bull, 2006. 32 Suppl 1: p. S44-63.

[26] Couture, S.M., E.L. Granholm, and S.C. Fish, A path model investigation of neurocognition, theory of mind, social competence, negative symptoms and real-world functioning in schizophrenia. Schizophr Res, 2011. 125(2-3): p. 152-60.

[27] Mancuso, F., et al., Social cognition in psychosis: multidimensional structure, clinical correlates, and relationship with functional outcome. Schizophr Res, 2011. 125(2-3): p. 143-51.

[28] Wolf, F., M. Brune, and H.J. Assion, Theory of mind and neurocognitive functioning in patients with bipolar disorder. Bipolar Disord, 2010. 12(6): p. 657-66.

[29] Lahera, G., et al., Theory of mind deficit in bipolar disorder: is it related to a previous history of psychotic symptoms? Psychiatry Res, 2008. 161(3): p. 309-17.

[30] Peron, J., et al., Are dopaminergic pathways involved in theory of mind? A study in Parkinson's disease. Neuropsychologia, 2009. 47(2): p. 406-14.

[31] Langdon, R., et al., Mentalising, executive planning and disengagement in schizophrenia. Cognitive Neuropsychiatry, 2001. 6(2): p. 81-108.

[32] Pickup, G.J., Relationship between Theory of Mind and executive function in schizophrenia: a systematic review. Psychopathology, 2008. 41(4): p. 206-13.

[33] Bassett, D.S., et al., Hierarchical organization of human cortical networks in health and schizophrenia. J Neurosci, 2008. 28(37): p. 9239-48.
[34] Cohen, J., A power Primer. Psychological Bulletin, 1992. 112(1): p. 155-59.
[35] Lysaker, P.H., et al., Metacognition in schizophrenia: associations with multiple assessments of executive function. J Nerv Ment Dis, 2008. 196(5): p. 384-9.
[36] Vaskinn, A., et al., Emotion perception and learning potential: mediators between neurocognition and social problem-solving in schizophrenia? J Int Neuropsychol Soc, 2008. 14(2): p. 279-88.
[37] Rocca, P., et al., Exploring the role of face processing in facial emotion recognition in schizophrenia. Acta Neuropsychiatrica, 2009. 21: p. 292–300.
[38] Brune, M., Emotion recognition, 'theory of mind,' and social behavior in schizophrenia. Psychiatry Res, 2005. 133(2-3): p. 135-47.
[39] Langdon, R., et al., Disturbed communication in schizophrenia: the role of poor pragmatics and poor mind-reading. Psychol Med, 2002. 32(7): p. 1273-84.
[40] Majorek, K., et al., "Theory of mind" and executive functioning in forensic patients with schizophrenia. J Forensic Sci, 2009. 54(2): p. 469-73.
[41] Lancaster, R.S., et al., Social cognition and neurocognitive deficits in schizophrenia. J Nerv Ment Dis, 2003. 191(5): p. 295-9.
[42] Bailey, P.E. and J.D. Henry, Separating component processes of theory of mind in schizophrenia. Br J Clin Psychol, 2010. 49(Pt 1): p. 43-52.
[43] Bell, M., et al., Neurocognition, social cognition, perceived social discomfort, and vocational outcomes in schizophrenia. Schizophr Bull, 2009. 35(4): p. 738-47.
[44] Cohen, A.S., et al., Specific cognitive deficits and differential domains of social functioning impairment in schizophrenia. Schizophr Res, 2006. 81(2-3): p. 227-38.
[45] Ikebuchi, E., Social skills and social and nonsocial cognitive functioning in schizophrenia. Journal of Mental Health, 2007. 16(5): p. 581-94.
[46] Mazza, M., et al., Pragmatic language and theory of mind deficits in people with schizophrenia and their relatives. Psychopathology, 2008. 41(4): p. 254-63.
[47] Tsoi, D.T., et al., Humour experience in schizophrenia: relationship with executive dysfunction and psychosocial impairment. Psychol Med, 2008. 38(6): p. 801-10.
[48] Frith, C., Theory of Mind in Schizophrenia, in The Cognitive Neuropsychology of Schizophrenia., A. David and J. Cutting, Editors. 1992, Lawrence Erlbaum: Hove. p. 147-161.
[49] Penn, D.L., et al., Social cognition in schizophrenia. Psychol Bull, 1997. 121(1): p. 114-32.
[50] Addington, J., H. Saeedi, and D. Addington, Facial affect recognition: a mediator between cognitive and social functioning in psychosis? Schizophr Res, 2006. 85(1-3): p. 142-50.
[51] Addington, J., H. Saeedi, and D. Addington, Influence of social perception and social knowledge on cognitive and social functioning in early psychosis. Br J Psychiatry, 2006 b. 189: p. 373-8.

[52] Koutsouleris, N., et al., Neuroanatomical correlates of executive dysfunction in the at-risk mental state for psychosis. Schizophr Res, 2010. 123(2-3): p. 160-74.
[53] Schnieder, T.P. and A.J. Dwork, Searching for neuropathology: gliosis in schizophrenia. Biol Psychiatry, 2011. 69(2): p. 134-9.

6

Directions in Research into Response Selection Slowing in Schizophrenia

D.P. McAllindon[1,2] and P.G. Tibbo[2]
[1]*National Research Council Canada, Institute for Biodiagnostics (Atlantic)*
[2]*Department of Psychiatry, Dalhousie University Canada*

1. Introduction

People with schizophrenia experience many types of symptoms and a particularly difficult type are cognitive. Cognitive deficits are relevant to prognosis (Green, 1996; Green, Kern, Braff & Mintz, 2000) and improvement in cognitive skills may produce gains in emotional, physical, social and vocational adaptation (Matza et al., 2006). Response selection slowing is perhaps the most straightforward way to show a cognitive deficit in schizophrenia and has a long history in schizophrenia research. Response selection plays a role in virtually any task that requires a motor response; thus it is important to understand it fully in the context of schizophrenia to allow appropriate and valid interpretation of other cognitive tasks. Adding to its importance is that response selection may also be an endophenotype of schizophrenia. This paper will summarize recent results in neuroimaging of response selection in schizophrenia. As well, the best test of our understanding of the deficit in response selection slowing in schizophrenia will be through simulation, so progress in computational models using neural networks will also be examined.

This chapter will begin by summarizing the long history of research in response selection slowing in schizophrenia. It will then proceed with a description of various neuroimaging techniques that are used in the studies that will be discussed. Following that, landmark studies in response selection in healthy people will be summarized followed by the discussion of studies in response selection in schizophrenia. The next-to-last section will highlight some research in simulation that show promise in modeling the differences in response selection in people with schizophrenia before ending with a concluding paragraph.

2. History of response selection slowing in schizophrenia

The prototypical response selection task is choice reaction time (RT) with RT being the measured variable. Whereas simple RT tasks require the same response to any stimulus, choice RT requires a decision among a choice of responses dependent on the stimulus. The modality (auditory, visual, tactile) makes a difference in the RT, with auditory being faster than visual (Naito et al., 2000), as well as stimulus-response compatibility, where responses that are more compatible are faster, and the preparatory interval (period of time before the stimulus) where a longer RT generally results from a longer preparatory interval. Studies of response selection almost invariably require a series of trials, and the order of trials and mix (regular/irregular) of preparatory intervals can lead to effects on reaction times which have been exploited in various ways. Variables of interest include median RT, measures of the distribution of reaction times (e.g. interquartile range), mistakes (incorrect response to stimulus), errors of omission (no response to a stimulus) and errors of commission (responding without a stimulus).

A slowing in visual or auditory RT was demonstrated in early schizophrenia research (for a review, see Wells & Kelley, 1922). Investigation of response selection in schizophrenia was extensive through the middle decades of the 20th century (see Nuechterlein (1977), for a review), and many versions of RT tasks were developed in pursuit of an objective test for schizophrenia (e.g. Huston, Shakow & Riggs, 1937); however, the results were never specific enough to be used with confidence for individuals. A strength of these early studies is that when they were completed, neuroleptic and antipsychotic drugs were not available, so patients participating in these studies were drug-free. However, the diagnosis of schizophrenia has evolved over time. The Diagnostic and Statistical Manual of Mental Disorders (DSM) wasn't introduced until 1952 and dramatically revised and accepted in the 1980s, so modern studies use a somewhat different sample.

Similar to measures of more complex cognitive functions, the response selection deficits in schizophrenia are related to poor outcome. Studies by Zahn and Carpenter and Cancro et al. in the 1970s correlated longer RT with increased hospitalization for schizophrenia (Zahn & Carpenter, 1978; Cancro, Sutton, Kerr & Sugarman, 1971). Silverstein et al. included auditory simple RT in a study involving several other common neurocognitive tests (Silverstein, Schenkel, Valone & Nuernberger, 1998). They found that the presence of an error of commission predicted reduced performance at the end of training of individuals with schizophrenia.

More recently, Ngan and Liddle studied reaction times in populations with schizophrenia and found (negative) correlation between disorganization and negative symptoms with simple RT in persistent illness populations, and (negative) correlation between disorganization symptoms with choice RT in the same population (Ngan & Liddle, 2000). Another recent study (Pellizzer & Stephane, 2007) found that mean RT in a 2-choice RT task did not predict mean reaction time (RT) in a 4-choice RT task in people with schizophrenia, whereas as it did for healthy controls. They suggested that this indicates that the slowing in schizophrenia from increased choices is a different process from the slowing in healthy persons.

Response selection slowing in schizophrenia could also be important due to its heritability. Reaction time has been shown to be one of the most heritable cognitive tasks. A twin study looking at both simple and choice RT found 64% and 62% heritability respectively at 16 years of age (Rijsdijk, Vernon & Boomsma, 1998). Another twin study also found 64% heritability for choice RT (Wright et al., 2001). This is higher than working memory tasks (below 50% in Wright et al., 2001). As well, RT has been shown to be weakly but reliably correlated with IQ, with estimates of between -0.2 and -0.4 (Rijsdijk et al., 1998; Wright et al., 2001).

The heritability of response selection would be important if we can show a difference between people with schizophrenia, first-degree relatives of schizophrenia and healthy volunteers using neuroimaging. Schizophrenia has a sizable genetic loading, but there has been limited progress in identifying suspect genes for schizophrenia. One reason argued for limited progress in genetic analysis is that schizophrenia may not be a single disease (e.g. Hallmeyer et al., 2005). Subsequently, active research programs are on to identify endophenotypes (Braff, 2007). Where phenotypes are the outward, visible expression of the genotype, endophenotypes are an intermediate expression of the genotype that must be measured rather than being obviously visible. Endophenotypes are regarded as closer to the genetic variation than the phenotype, and thus endophenotypes of schizophrenia may be more amenable to genetic analysis than the phenotype. Endophenotypes should show measurable differences between people with schizophrenia and healthy volunteers, as well as being heritable. Therefore, response selection is an excellent candidate for an endophenotype as it is strongly heritable and is measurably different.

It is important to point out that although choice RT seems like a simple paradigm, it in fact involves many complications because of the serial presentation for neuroimaging. It seems that there are many unconscious operations that may be involved, as well as attention, and the many different details of paradigms can affect these. Some of these unconscious operations must include interval timing and recognizing patterns. For example, the fMRI study by Praamstra et al. (2006) investigates interval timing using a serial choice RT task (Praamstra et al., 2006), and several studies in schizophrenia have examined procedural learning with a serial choice RT paradigm (Zedkova et al., 2006; Woodward et al., 2007). These complications can introduce difficulties in interpreting results, especially since, as we have seen with various ACC activations, these activations can happen at different times post-stimulus and may be involved in different processes of the task.

3. Neuroimaging studies of response selection

Research into response selection slowing has been revived by advances in neuroimaging. Neuroimaging offers possibilities to identify where and when the deficits in schizophrenia arise in the response selection process. A first step is to understand the process in healthy people. Neuroimaging studies of response selection have been reported using the full suite of imaging techniques including PET (e.g. Iacoboni et al., 1996; Naito et al., 2000), EEG (e.g. Mulert et al., 2003), fMRI (Jiang and Kanwisher, 2003; Winterer et al., 2002) and MEG (Thoma et al., 2006).

3.1 Neuroimaging techniques

There have been many neuroimaging techniques employed in the study of response selection. To appreciate the literature, an understanding of these techniques is important. The techniques are described briefly below.

Electroencephalography (EEG) was first used on humans by Hans Berger in 1924. It measures electrical potentials on the scalp using a number of electrodes, e.g. International 10-20 system for clinical use has 19 electrodes plus a reference; research systems typically have more electrodes. The potentials are created by changing ionic current flows in populations of neurons (hundreds of thousands to millions) and are in the range of plus and minus 100 μV. Each electrode records the potential across time at a high resolution (milliseconds). EEG is often used to record event-related potentials (ERPs) by repeating events many times. ERPs are created from raw EEG signals by cutting each session into individual events, synchronizing the events according to an external signal (either stimulus or response) and averaging them together. This eliminates noise and allows the detection of peaks and valleys that line up with the stimulus or the response, depending on which is chosen as the reference (stimulus-locked or response-locked). The transmission of the electric potentials through the head is complicated and difficult to model, and this limits the ability to determine the spatial source of the EEG signals. EEG equipment is cheap compared to the other techniques described and can be done on almost anyone.

Magnetoencephalography (MEG) resembles EEG, and can be analyzed using the same methods, but measures magnetic potentials around the head instead of electrical potentials. Instead of electrodes contacting the scalp, it uses magnetic potentiometers and gradiometers that do not have to contact the scalp. The magnetic fields are very, very small (pT) and are easily overwhelmed by environmental noise such as cars passing by on the street, or elevators moving within the building, so MEG machines must be kept in very well shielded rooms. The potentiometers are based on SQUIDS - supercooled quantum interference devices. The magnetic potentials transmit through the head in a much more well-defined manner than the electrical potentials and many more potentiometers may be used, so MEG provides the potential for spatial resolution of sources to within 5 mm as well as millisecond time resolution like EEG (although the ability of MEG to detect and spatialize signals from deep within the brain is in question). MEG equipment is quite expensive, but its advantages and the fact that almost anyone can be scanned with MEG make it a desirable neuroimaging technique.

Functional magnetic resonance imaging (fMRI) uses magnetic resonance imaging sequences that are sensitized to blood flow in the brain. Blood flows more to active areas of the brain, to maintain energy to run the neural electrical interactions and biochemical reactions. The most common technique is BOLD (blood oxygen level dependent), demonstrated by Ogawa in 1990 (Ogawa et al., 1990). Blood oxygen level increases with neural activity as oxygen-laden blood rushes in to areas of high activity. Deoxygenated blood has a different magnetic susceptibility than oxygenated blood, which creates small changes in the local magnetic environment that can be measured with the magnetic resonance imaging scanner. As the changes are small, the activation is detected statistically, usually by comparing the measured signal with the expected signal under a general linear model framework. Cognitive tasks are analyzed using block designs as used in PET studies (fMRI's predecessor), or with event-related designs that are more similar to EEG or MEG paradigms. As the measurement of neural activity is indirect - through blood flow changes and then magnetic environment changes - physiological changes unrelated to cognitive activity can also affect the signal measured by fMRI. The hemodynamic response is the shape of the measured response to instantaneous neural activity. The shape of the hemodynamic response has been measured in various specific situations and brain areas and found to be roughly consistent between people and brain areas, and to add up roughly linearly to a sequence of events. The hemodynamic response has a delay of a few seconds, a rise up to a plateau and then a drop back to equilibrium. In all, the hemodynamic response can last 20 seconds before return to equilibrium in response to a brief neural event. The shape is often assumed in the analysis with only amplitude varied, though some analysis techniques do not depend on knowledge of this shape. fMRI is able to provide spatial localization to within a few mm, but has poor time resolution as a result of the hemodynamic response, although clever methods have been developed to measure events to a finer time resolution.

Positron emission tomography (PET) uses radioactive tracers that are injected into the subjects. The radioactive tracers emit positrons that give off gamma rays (photons) that can be detected on the outside of the machine when the positrons interact with matter. The gamma rays travel in approximately opposite directions after they are created and the machine notes gamma rays that arrive on opposite sides of the detector at approximately the same time. The machine can then trace the pair of gamma rays back to identify where they originated. In a session, many of these events must be counted and traced back to determine the levels of radioactivity in the body. Different radiotracers can be injected that will bind to different functional processes in the body, allowing many different types of functions to be imaged. The most common tracer in neuroimaging is fluorodeoxyglucose (FDG), a sugar that performs the same functions biologically as glucose. In the brain, FDG is taken up more by active cells, leading to increased radioactivity in active parts of the brain. The measurement is referred to as regional cerebral blood flow (rCBF). However, the use of ionizing radiation limits performing multiple scans on the same individual. As well, the radioisotopes take some time to reach their destination in the body (~ 1 hour with FDG), and time to count, limiting the kinds of cognitive tasks that can studied. PET was developed before fMRI and was used for cognitive studies in the 80s and 90s, but is not widely used for these purposes anymore.

3.2 Neuroimaging studies of response selection in healthy controls

The first neuroimaging applications to response selection used PET (Taylor et al., 1994; Iacoboni et al., 1996). Taylor's study found that increased rCBF in the cingulate gyrus correlated with faster reaction time. Iacoboni used a choice RT task with a visual stimulus with button response from either hand (stimulus-response compatible) or reversed response (incompatible) and found increased rCBF in bilateral superior parietal lobules with the incompatible task. Another study by Naito et al. (2000) looked at simple RT to stimuli in various modalities in healthy volunteers using positron emission tomography (PET) (Naito et al., 2000). They found that in all modalities, the reaction time was negatively correlated with activation in a part of the anterior cingulate cortex (ACC) (See Figure 1).

Mulert and colleagues looked at choice RT to an auditory stimulus using electroencephalography (EEG) and low resolution electromagnetic tomography (LORETA - a method to determine spatial location of electrical sources) and found a similar relation between current density in ACC, RT, and error rate (Mulert et al., 2003). Mulert and colleagues used the same paradigm and analysis to compare people with schizophrenia to healthy controls (Mulert et al., 2001) and first-episode schizophrenia (Gallinat et al., 2002). These results will be highlighted in the next section.

fMRI has frequently been used to investigate response selection. In some cases, a choice RT task is used as a control and such was the case with Jansma and colleagues (2000). Jansma's study, which was intended to look at learning, included choice RT to a visual stimulus in healthy volunteers and found ACC activity among other activations, although they did not attempt to correlate RT to degree of ACC activation (Jansma et al., 2000).

Another study examined choice RT with a visual stimulus in healthy volunteers using event-related fMRI (Winterer et al., 2002) and found the same negative correlation between activity in ACC and RT (see Figure 1) as had been found by their group earlier in auditory choice RT using EEG (Mulert et al., 2001).

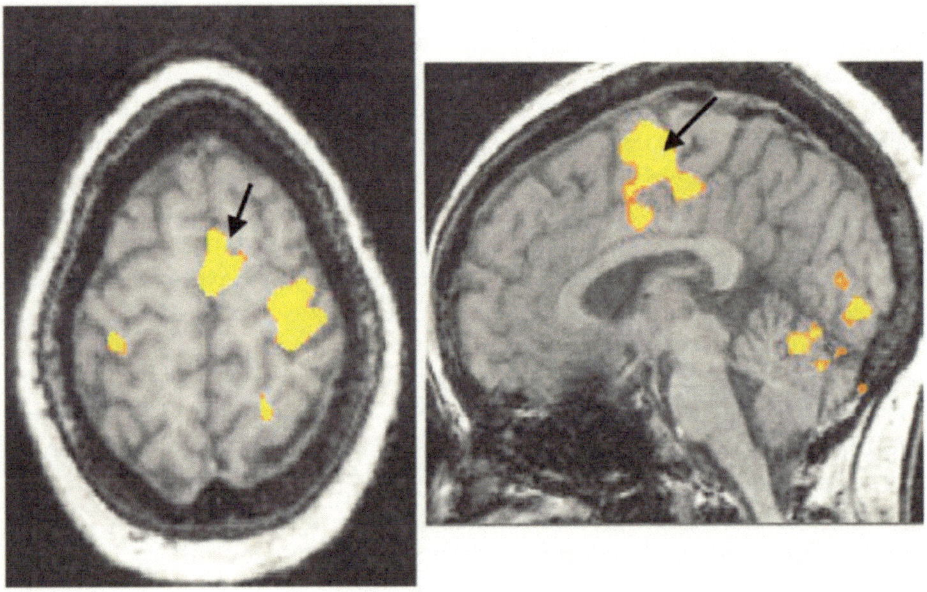

Fig. 1. Results from Winterer et al. (2001) showing activation in ACC/SMA from event-related visual 2-choice reaction time task. Reprinted with permission.

The fact that ACC activation in a response selection task in healthy populations has been consistently found by different researchers using different imaging techniques and different paradigms makes it a robust finding. There is a conflict about ACC function between theories of selection-for-action (Posner & DiGirolamo, 1994) and conflict monitoring (Carter et al., 2000), but these differing roles may be resolved by findings that ACC is a heterogeneous functional area (Swick & Jovanovic, 2002; Vogt et al., 1992; Picard & Strick 1996), and that ACC activity is seen at different times during the response, namely early (~ 130 ms post-stimulus) (Mulert et al., 2001) and late (~240 ms, 360 ms, 390 ms and 414 ms post-stimulus) (Winterer et al., 2001).

Another task that provides some insight into this controversy is the Attention Network Task (ANT) developed by Fan (2001) to investigate different aspects of attention: namely alerting, orienting and executing. An event-related fMRI study of the ANT task identified ACC activity only during the executive aspect (Fan et al., 2005). The study compared results from one aspect with results from another, so any activation that is common in the aspects of the ANT task is not identified as a component of a particular aspect. Thus, the activation during the executive phase is most likely the late activation of ACC connected with performance (conflict) monitoring, and early activation of ACC in the response selection is not identified.

Several other fMRI studies have focused on various aspects of response selection in healthy populations. Dassonville et al. (2001) looked at the effect of stimulus-response compatibility at 2 levels - set-level and element-level (Dassonville et al., 2001). Set-level changes the set of stimulus and response characteristics (using spatial versus symbolic stimulus in this experiment), whereas element level changes only the mapping between stimulus and response (such as reversing responses in the Iacoboni et al. (1996) task, or in the Dassonville experiment, direct or counter-clockwise mapping). In this study, 4 conditions were compared in 11 regions-of-interest. Element-level changes produced more activation in pre-supplementary motor area, dorsal and ventral premotor areas and parietal areas, and activation was lateralized to the right hemisphere. Set-level changes produced more activation in the same areas plus inferior frontal gyri, anterior cingulate, cingulate motor areas and superior temporal lobe, and activations were lateralized to the left hemisphere (see Figure 2). These results apply to changes in stimulus-response compatibility of the tasks, and the differences between the 3 sets in Figure 2 show the effect of set, element, and set and element level changes.

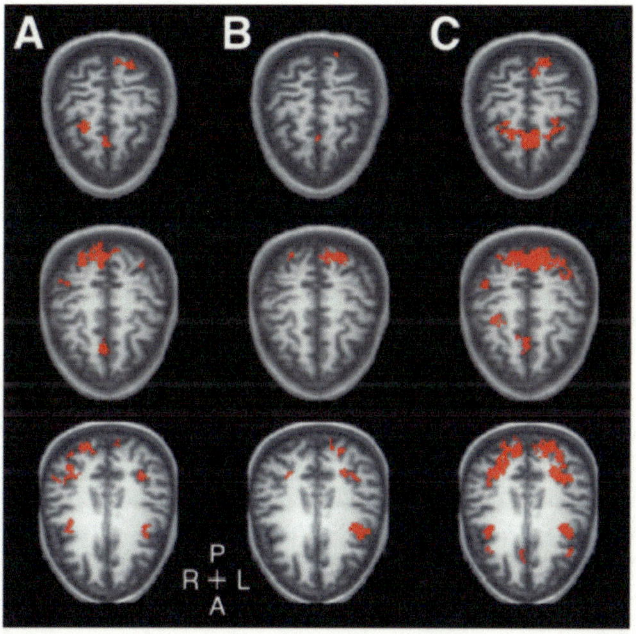

Fig. 2. Spatially congruent activation at three different anatomic levels in the (A) spatial/ccw, (B) symbolic/direct, and (C) symbolic/ccw tasks (A-B: set and element; B-C: element; A-C: set level changes). From Dassonville et al, 2001. Reprinted with permission.

A set of studies of response selection investigated commonality of functional activations with domain of stimulus (auditory, somatosensory, visual) and with perceptual processes (Jiang and Kanwisher, 2003; Jiang and Kanwisher, 2003a; Schumacher et al., 2003). The first study used a 4-choice perceptual decision task in visual, auditory and verbal domains to show common neural substrates of response selection with stimulus modality. These were found across bilateral parietal and frontal regions. The second study compared perception and response selection tasks and found common activation between them in all the ROIs investigated, a contradictory finding to the behavioural finding that response selection is a unitary process subject to dual task interference whereas perceptual processing can carry on in parallel. Schumacher and colleagues investigated the commonality of response selection between spatial and nonspatial stimuli and found a dissociation of areas. The conflicts between these findings were discussed by Schumacher and Jiang (Schumacher & Jiang, 2003), and although they can provide an explanation for the seemingly divergent results, the process provides an interesting lesson in the limitations of interpreting results from a single study; namely, to be careful how generally you interpret the results from a single task.

An interesting recent paper investigated trial-by-trial variation of RT using fMRI (Yarkoni et al., 2010). The authors describe the analysis of a set of results combined from several different studies of different tasks. All of the tasks were significantly more complex than choice RT with significantly longer reaction times. However, even with the use of different tasks, a set of areas was identified whose activity varied with the reaction time (time-on-task), and another set whose delay in activity correlated with reaction time (temporal shift). Areas showing time-on-task correlation would seem to be directly involved in the processes that vary in length to create variable RTs, whereas areas showing temporal shift would be areas that are activated following the time-on-task areas. An enormous set of regions was identified with the different effects roughly spatially-segregated. The time-on-task areas included frontoparietal and thalamic, whereas temporal shift were strongest in somatomotor, visual, cerebellar and posterior midline cortical regions. These results help to show the temporal sequence of activation of areas, and which areas are most responsible for varying RT. That this temporal sequence can be seen in fMRI results is very significant and provides motivation to attempt this type of breakdown in studies of schizophrenia. We will see alternate ways to approach this temporal sequence issue using EEG and MEG in the next section.

Choice RT has even been investigated in connection with white matter pathways supporting visuospatial attention (Tuch et al., 2005). This study used diffusion tensor imaging, a technique of MRI, to measure the fractional anisotropy (FA - a measure of orientation coherence of water self-diffusion indicating health of white matter pathways) of white matter pathways in the brain and found a positive correlation between FA and choice RT in several different pathways associated with visual processing. It would be very interesting to perform such a study in people with schizophrenia to look for a similar correlation between FA and choice RT.

A MEG study of response selection has also been reported (Thoma et al., 2006). The study concentrated on the timing of various identifiable steps in the response selection process for simple and 2-choice RT tasks. These were visual - identified by a magnetic dipole in contralateral calcarine cortex; motor – identified by a magnetic dipole in pre-central gyrus immediately prior to the response; and somatosensory – identified by a magnetic dipole in post-central gyrus immediately following the response (see Figure 3). The behavioural response occurred between the motor and somatosensory dipoles. Visual-Motor Integration (VMI) time was calculated as the difference between the visual dipole and the motor dipole.

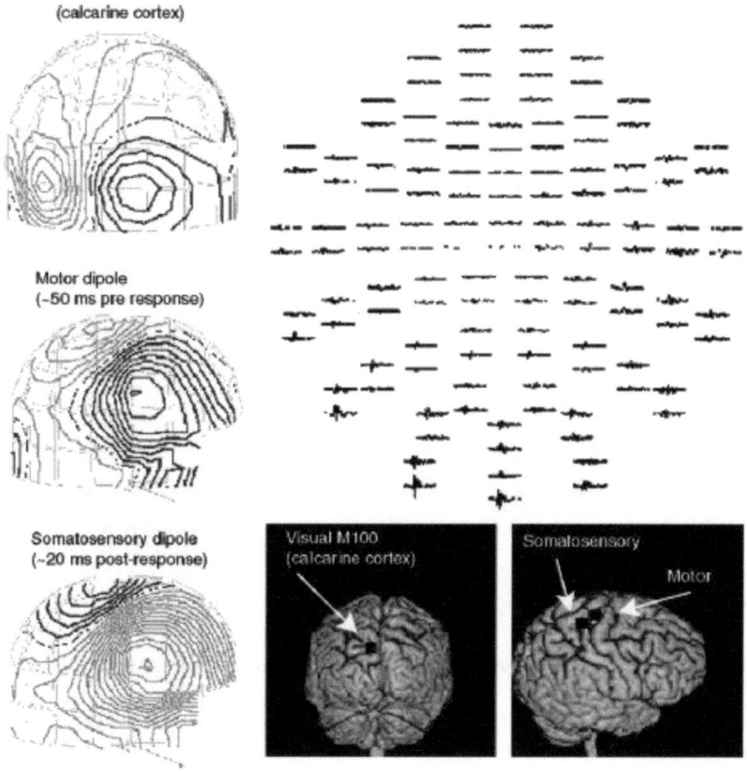

Fig. 3. A right-visual hemifield stimulus presentation with left hand response results in MEG data as shown. This figure contains a field pattern, contour map for each dipole, and localization for each of visual, motor, and somatosensory dipoles. From Thoma et al, 2006. Reprinted with permission.

The visual stimulus was a circular checkerboard presented briefly (50 ms) in left or right hemisphere and four conditions were used - right-only response, left-only, ipsilateral response and contralateral response. MEG and RT data were correlated with scores on Raven's Advanced Progressive Matrices and fluctuating asymmetry, a measure of developmental instability. Significant correlations included a negative correlation between the VMI time and RAPM score (smaller VMI time with higher score) and a positive correlation between the visual response latency and RAPM score. The results show that the varying reaction times arise primarily between the visual and motor dipoles. Although this is quite a broad breakdown of the temporal sequence and a finer scale would be useful, similar studies in people with schizophrenia would be useful to identify where and when neural processes are different from healthy people.

Another neuroimaging technique that is relevant in the context of animal studies is single neuron recording. Animals such as monkeys can be trained to perform various forms of choice RT tasks, and modern electrodes and surgical implantation techniques allows recording from conscious animals while they perform these tasks. The advantage of such recordings is the specificity and time resolution. Prior knowledge is used to determine likely places to implant the electrodes to obtain a response for the particular cognitive task being investigated. In recent years, single-cell recording of awake monkeys performing a visual discrimination task has identified areas that may be involved in the decisions (Roitman & Schadlen, 2002; Schall, 2002). By correlating the rate of rise of activity in implanted areas with the behavioural decision time, areas in the middle temporal lobe, lateral intraparietal area in extrastriate cortex, the frontal eye field and superior colliculus have been identified. These results were specific to the task requiring a visual response (saccade) as well as a visual stimulus, so involvement of areas such as frontal eye field and superior colliculus is probably not relevant to a motor response, but middle temporal lobe and laterial intraparietal area could be more generally involved for any response.

In summary, response selection has been investigated for some time in healthy populations to aid in a better understanding of basic cognitive functioning. More sophisticated neuroimaging techniques and methodologies have allowed further refinement of the spatial and temporal sequencing of this key cognitive function., but there are unresolved questions about the temporal sequencing of functional areas involved in response selection.

3.3 Neuroimaging studies of response selection in schizophrenia

Several neuroimaging studies of response selection have looked specifically at individuals with schizophrenia (Mulert et al., 2001; Gallinat et al., 2002; Woodward et al., 2009; McAllindon et al., 2009; Luck et al., 2006; Luck et al., 2009). Other studies have used simple RT as a paradigm in people with schizophrenia (Barch et al., 2003).

The studies by Mulert and Gallinat were similar to each other and used EEG and an auditory choice RT paradigm. Mulert studied a population with chronic schizophrenia and Gallinat looked at first-episode psychosis. Both studies reached a similar conclusion that an area roughly identified as anterior cingulate cortex showed a lower current density in performing the task in people with schizophrenia (See Figures 4 and 5). It should be noted that these EEG studies concentrated on a time about 100 ms post-stimulus that may be a different function (selection-for-action) than activation in the ACC that has been identified at later times (conflict monitoring) (Winterer et al., 2002).

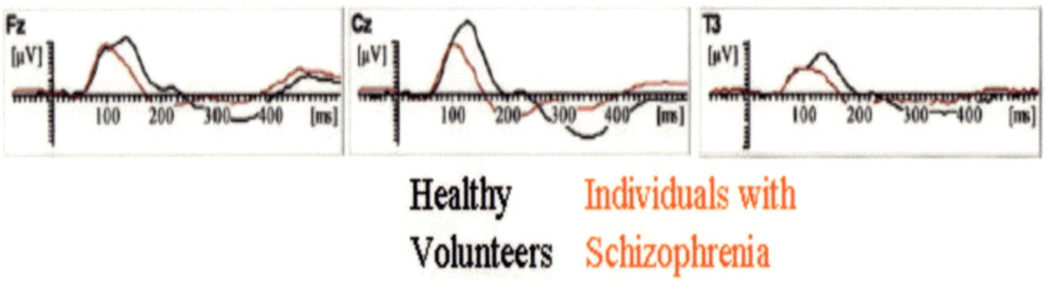

Fig. 4. Selected ERP grand averages comparing healthy volunteers (black) to individuals with schizophrenia (red). From Mulert et al., 2001. (Grand Average is average of all subjects' ERPs.) Reprinted with permission.

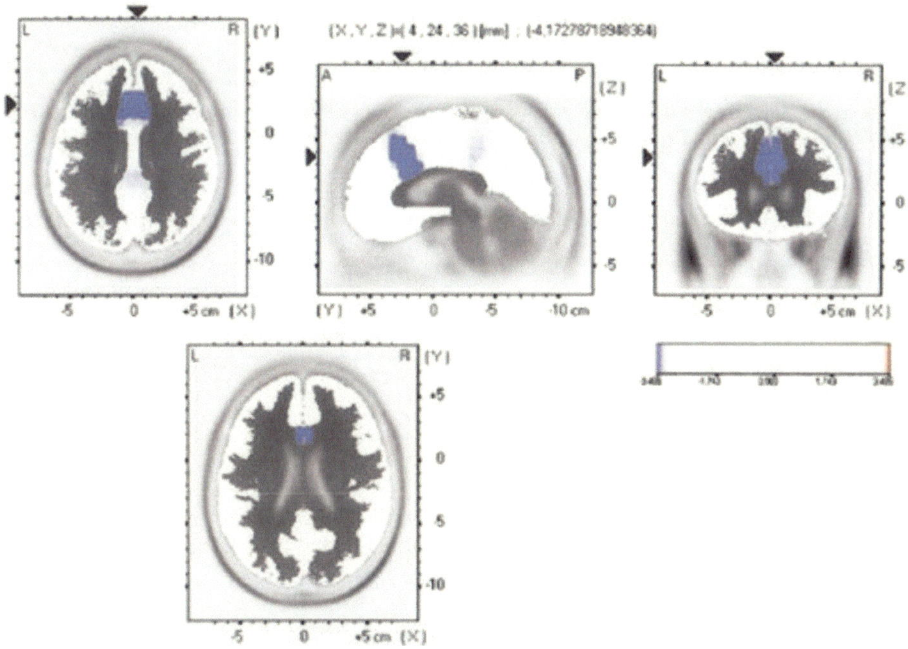

Fig. 5. LORETA results from ERP recordings showing reduction in current amplitude during auditory choice reaction time task. From Gallinat et al., 2002. Reprinted with permission.

Mulert proceeded to perform 2 further studies of response selection slowing to help explain the earlier findings. One possible explanation for the function of this early, ACC-related task is effort or degree of engagement with the task. This theory was investigated by Mulert et al. (2005) who were able to correlate ACC activation and RT with the self-reported effort on the task (Mulert et al., 2005) (See Figures 6 and 7). This is a very interesting explanation since a major confound with cognitive tasks on individuals with schizophrenia is whether the results are biased by their involvement with the task. The early ACC activity may actually be a neural sign of the degree of engagement in a task by individuals with schizophrenia (and healthy volunteers).

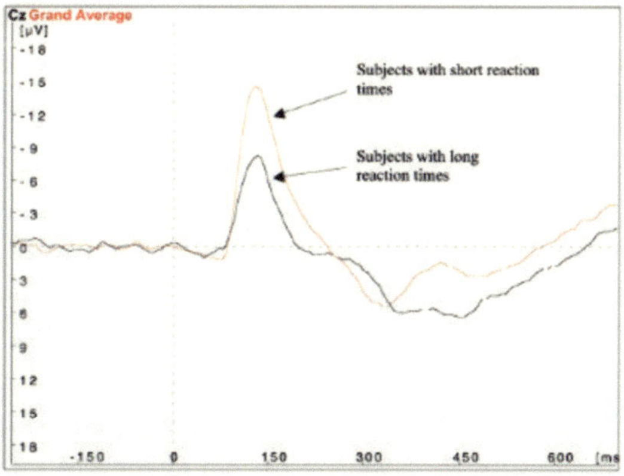

Fig. 6. Grand Average at Cz electrode for long and short reaction times. From Mulert et al., 2003. Reprinted with permission.

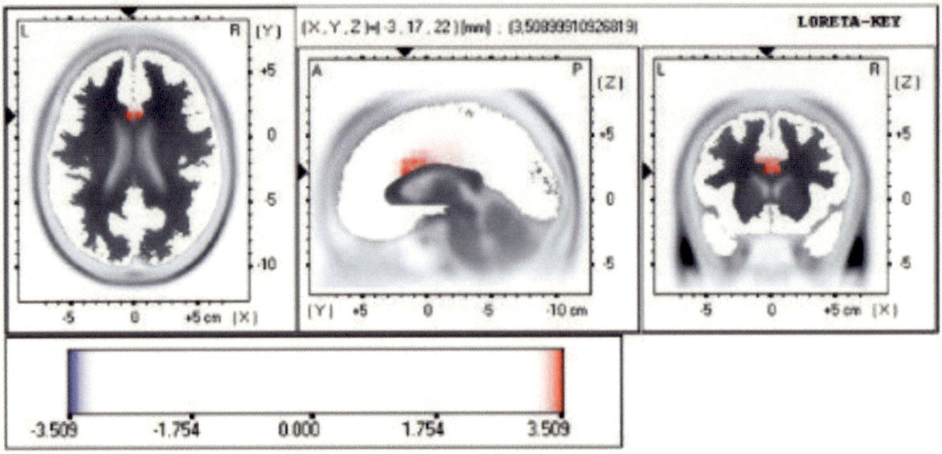

Fig. 7. LORETA results from ERP testing identifying area of increased current amplitude for short reaction times compared to long reaction times. From Mulert et al., 2003. Reprinted with permission.

Another of Mulert's studies (Mulert et al., 2003) (mentioned earlier) investigated the relation of error rate to RT and ACC activity, as the ACC has been suggested to be involved in performance monitoring (MacDonald et al., 2000). The results from this study found the expected relation between RT, error rate and current density in ACC. However, the timing of the tasks is important. The localization of performance monitoring functions to ACC has been shown by fMRI, which contains no time information. It would fit the evidence if the performance monitoring function of the ACC comes later than the response selection function, so that what we are seeing in response selection tasks is the early activation of ACC. Support for this idea also comes from neuroimaging of the ANT task, as discussed previously.

Luck has performed a series of EEG studies in an effort to localise when the cognitive deficit in response selection in people with schizophrenia occurs (Luck et al., 2006; Luck et al., 2009). The first of this series is reported in Luck et al. (2006), Experiment 1 and tries to identify if there is a deficit in speed of allocation of attention. It used the N2pc component as a marker of the time when perceptual processing becomes focused on a target item. The N2pc can be isolated laterally allowing it to be identified in a difference waveform. The task was to identify the side of a gap in a red or green square target in a sea of white squares against a dark grey background. In this, it was more complicated than a typical measure of response selection. The results showed a slowing of RT of about 150 ms in people with schizophrenia with a mean 800 ms RT for controls, but showed no difference in onset latency of the N2pc (see Figure 8). Both groups showed about 40 ms faster RT to red targets and about 50 ms less onset latency to red targets in the N2pc. Thus, there was no difference in speed of attention allocation.

The second experiment was a behavioural experiment that provided support for the interpretation of the first experiment. It used a variant of the Posner spatial cueing task that allowed a comparison of a behavioural measure of speed of allocation of attention between control and schizophrenia samples. The task was to report the identity of the letter in a circle of letters that is indicated by a marker before all letters are masked. By varying the time between the marker and the mask, the time to shift attention can be measured. Although there was a small increase in speed of attention of the schizophrenia sample of 102 ms versus 83 ms for controls that was marginally significant (p=0.053), this appeared to be entirely due to 4 outliers in the schizophrenia group. Luck et al. argue that these outliers are unrepresentative of the schizophrenia group as a whole and should be excluded. This behavioural measure would then agree with the neurimaging results showing no difference in speed of allocation of attention.

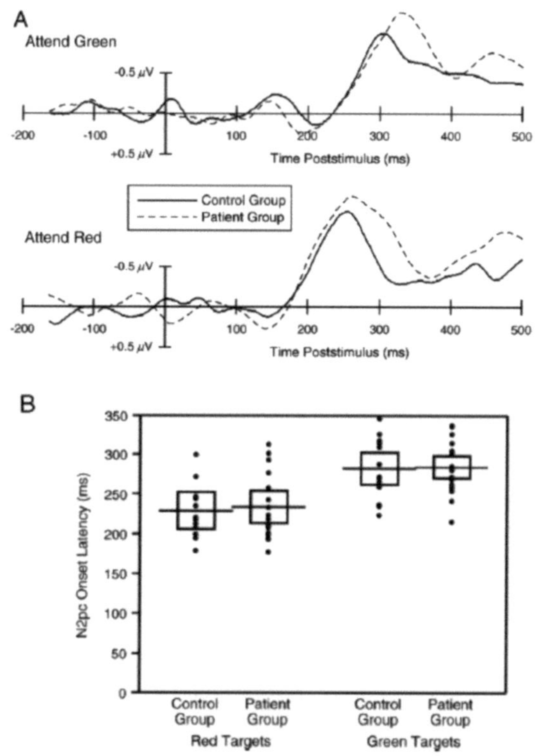

Fig. 8. (A) Grand average contralateral-minus-ipsilateral different waveforms from Luck et al. (2006)Experiment 1, averaged over the parietal, posterior occipital, lateral occipital, and posterior temporal electrode sites. Negative is plotted upward. (B) N2pc onset latency for each subject (filled circles), along with the mean and 95% confidence interval for each group. From Luck et al, 2006. Reprinted with permission.

A third experiment examined the categorization and response selection processes (Luck et al., 2009). This experiment used the P3 ERP and lateralized readiness potential (LRP) to identify when slowing occurred. The task was to respond with left or right hand depending on whether the stimulus was a letter or a digit. The response was reversed halfway through the session and the probabilities of letter or digit were adjusted throughout the sessions to produce a biased response for letters or digits or an equiprobable response. The P3 wave could be used to indicate the finish of perception and categorization and the LRP indicated the start of response preparation. Results showed no difference in latency of the P3 wave (part A of Figure 9) but a significant difference between controls and schizophrenia groups in latency of the LRP (part B of Figure 9). This indicates that the stage that was taking the most time was the response selection stage.

Several fMRI studies of response selection have been reported on people with schizophrenia. The earliest study used a simple RT task with a flashing checkerboard with a motor response to look at hemodynamic response function in people with schizophrenia (Barch et al., 2003). It found patients to be slower in RT, but to activate the same general areas with the same general hemodynamic response function. They used the finding to support the idea that differences in fMRI activation in people with schizophrenia are reflective of a real difference in activation rather than some difference in coupling between neural activity and the hemodynamic response function.

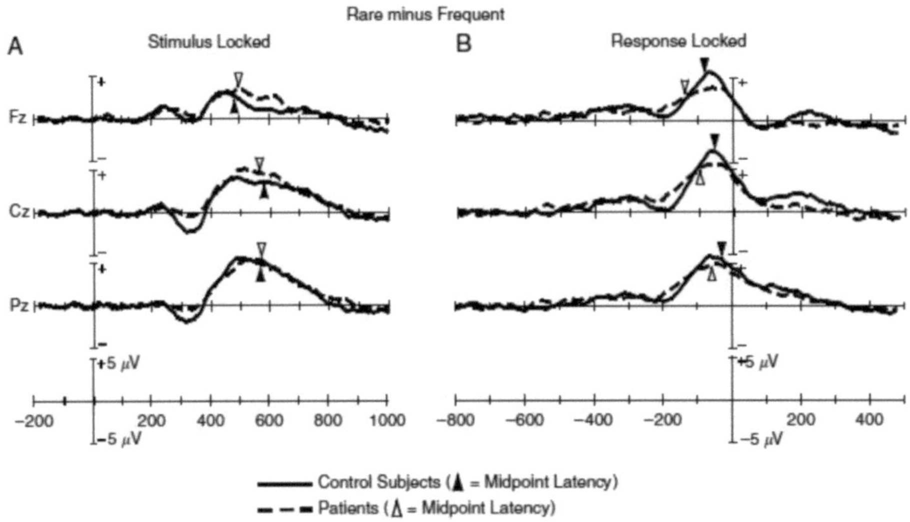

Fig. 9. Stimulus-locked (A) and response-locked (B) grand average ERP difference waveforms (rare minus frequent) from the patient and control groups at the frontal, central, and parietal midline electrode sites. Chart A shows the P3 wave and Chart B shows the LRP. Triangles indicate mean midpoint latency values. From Luck et al, 2009. Reprinted with permission.

Another study analyzed the data of a procedural learning study (Woodward et al., 2009). Although this study was set up to investigate procedural learning in schizophrenia, it included a block with random trials that could be analyzed versus fixation blocks. The task was a visual 4-choice spatially stimulus-response compatible task using 4 buttons on the dominant hand. The study included first-episode psychosis, chronic and first-degree unaffected sibling groups. The study found slower choice RT in all these groups compared to healthy controls, increased errors in patient groups, and increased BOLD activation in right dorsolateral prefrontal cortex (DLPFC, Brodmann Area 9) (see Figure 10). As well, a functional connectivity analysis using the right DLPFC area as a seed identified reduced connectivity in people with schizophrenia with many areas and found that connectivity between right DLPFC and right Brodmann area 40 correlated with RT in only patients, not controls. Overall, the results pointed towards choice RT fitting the criteria for an endophenotype.

Finally, another fMRI study used a difference between watching the visual stimuli and performing a motor response to remove visual activations and other common processes from the activation maps (McAllindon et al., 2009), and leave just the response selection and motor response processes. With a small sample size of 15 in chronic schizophrenia and healthy volunteer groups, the study found only a trend to lower activation in ACC in people with chronic schizophrenia, accompanied by an increase in RT.

In summary, response selection slowing has been investigated in people with schizophrenia with many different techniques and paradigms. A key future line of research is to understand when in the temporal sequence of cognitive processes the cognitive deficit appears in people with schizophrenia. Since spatial location of a deficit may in fact be in connectivity between functional areas in the brain, the temporal sequence may be the best clue to the deficit.

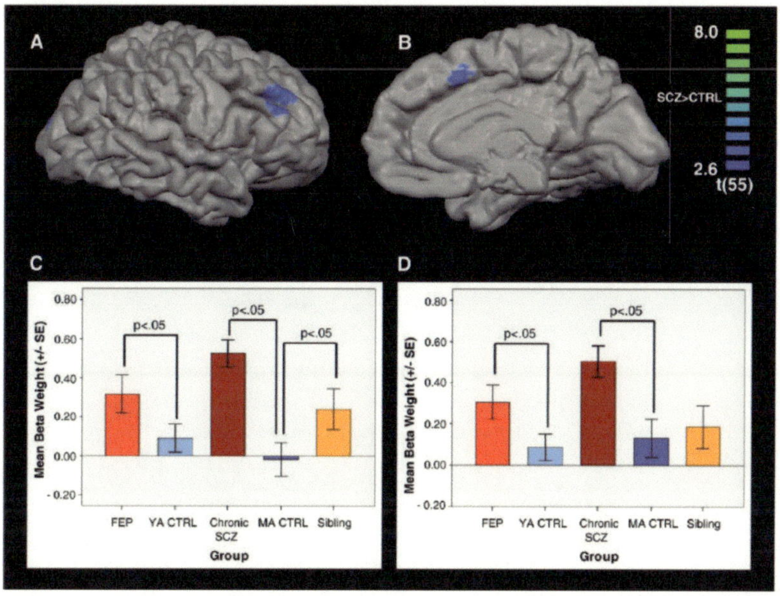

Fig. 10. Differences in brain activity between patients with schizophrenia, unaffected siblings, and healthy controls during choice reaction time task. Compared to controls, patients demonstrated greater activity during CRT blocks in right BA 9 (A) and right SMA (B). Activity in right BA 9 (C) and right SMA (D), in terms of task predictor beta weights. From Woodward et al, 2009. Reprinted with permission.

4. Models of response selection

Models of response selection have the potential to contribute greatly to the understanding of this process and how it can be affected by disease or neurological disorders. Specific theories can be developed and tested with reference to such models. Neuroimaging plays an important part in developing these models at the proper level to test theories of deficit.

There are many different types of models. A type that has been most researched is mathematical modelling. An early model of this type was Hicks' Law, which explained the dependence of reaction time on the number of choices:

$$\text{Mean RT} = K\log_2(n+1) \quad (1)$$

Where, K is a constant that changes for each individual, and
n is the number of choices

Various additions to the basic Hick's Law can account for the effect of frequency, the effect of sequence, the effect of discriminability and the effect of errors.

The most successful modern models are the Ornstein-Uhlenbeck diffusion model and the leaky competing accumulator model (Smith & Ratcliff, 2004.) Both models are for a 2-choice reaction time task and can predict most aspects of the RT distributions, including fast errors. In the leaky, competing accumulator model, 2 connected leaky accumulators gather evidence for their related response from the stimulus (see Figure 11). Accumulation is modelled as a stochastic process so that there can be variability in the RT results even when the stimulus is exactly the same, and so that mistakes can sometimes occur, as in behavioural results.

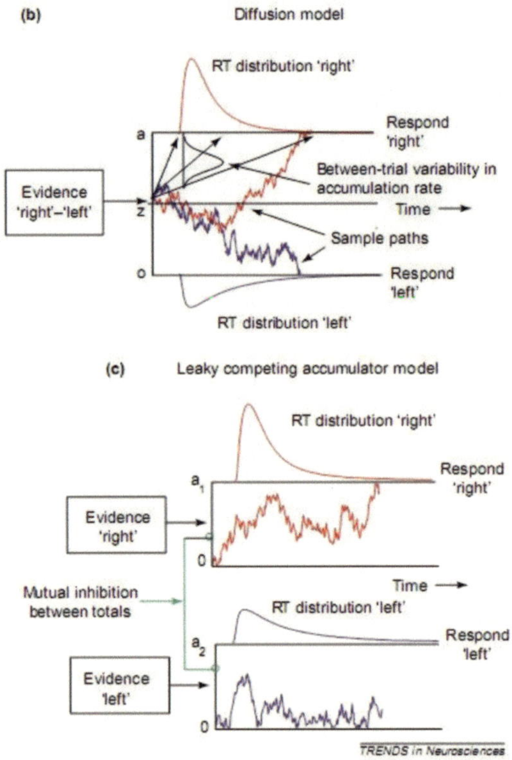

Fig. 11. Mathematical Models of Reaction Time (from Smith and Ratcliff, 2004) Reprinted with permission.

A simpler mathematical model is the linear ballistic accumulator model of Brown and Heathcote (Brown & Heathcote, 2008). This model uses linear rather than random walk accumulation with random starting levels in the accumulators. The model can successfully show the distribution of RT for multiple choice RTs, successfully repeat the pattern of correct and incorrect RTs, and has complete analytic solutions for multiple choice situations.

Another type of model is the computational model. These models are inspired by neural networks and take more or less biologically-principled views of the real neural networks that can be configured to response selection tasks, or whatever cognitive function is being modelled. These models can provide insight on the various levels at which they are modelled, and show the most promise in testing theories of deficit because of their biological relevance. Based on what has been discovered about the neurophysiology of the visual saccade task in monkeys, biologically-plausible neuronal simulations have been built that replicate real behavioural RT results (Wong & Wang, 2006; Lo & Wang, 2006). Wong's work modelled the basic task and they could use the model to show that the time integration in LIP neurons must be mediated by NMDA receptors rather than AMPA receptors. Lo and Wang's work was specifically trying to answer questions about the decision threshold in RT tasks and whether variability in the threshold could be modelled with a biophysically-based model. They found that a network including neocortex, basal ganglia and superior colliculus could perform the task, and that the basal ganglia was primarily responsible for the decision threshold. Although the work is specific to the visual saccade task, one can imagine a similar network being developed for a RT task involving manual response.

Lo and Wang's model is very suggestive for RT results in schizophrenia because of the connections of mid-brain dopamine neurons with neurons in the caudate (part of the basal ganglia). If a circuit involving the caudate is involved in setting decision threshold, it could be influenced by dopamine levels (Kiana, Shanks & Shadlen, 2006). We know that dopamine is implicated in schizophrenia, and the above model results suggest a mechanism how the abnormal dopamine levels could affect reaction times.

5. Conclusions

Recent neuroimaging research into the response selection deficit in schizophrenia as summarized in this chapter shows promise to unravel the details of why people with schizophrenia have slower and more variable reaction times. This progress appears at many different levels, from behavioural studies identifying performance differences in people with schizophrenia, to a more detailed understanding of the neural processes involved in response selection from basic animal and human research, to finding particular processes and areas showing deficit in people with schizophrenia, to testing of theories in computational models. The approaches that break the task into stages to investigate when the deficit occurs offer promise in finding the deficit, and the increasing sophistication of models offers promise in being able to test theories of deficits. A detailed understanding of a relatively simple cognitive task such as choice reaction time will improve understanding of neuroimaging results of other cognitive tasks.

The promise of this research and understanding of response selection slowing and cognitive deficits in general is, of course, recovery. Rehabilitation programs can be developed to target specific deficits, and research into neural plasticity shows promise that effective rehabilitation programs can offer real hope of recovery. In addition, new medicines could be developed to target underlying physiological deficiencies. But it will be a long hard road yet to reach this promise.

6. References

Barch, D.M., Mathews, J.R., Buckner, R.L., Maccotta, L., Csernansky, J.G. & Snyder, A.Z. (2003). Hemodynamic responses in visual, motor, and somatosensory cortices in schizophrenia, *NeuroImage*, Vol. 20, No. 3, (December 2003), pp. 1884-1893

Braff, D.L., Freedman, R., Schork, N.J., & Gottesman, I.I. (2007). Deconstructing schizophrenia: An overview of the use of endophenotypes in order to understand a complex disorder. *Schizophrenia Bulletin*, Vol. 33, No. 1, (January 2007), pp. 21-32

Brown, S. D. & Heathcote, A. (2008). The simplest complete model of choice reaction time: Linear ballistic accumulation. *Cognitive Psychology*, Vol. 57, No. 3, (November 2008), pp. 153-178

Cancro, R. Sutton, S., Kerr, J. & Sugarman, A.A. (1971). Reaction time and prognosis in acute schizophrenia. *Journal of Nervous and Mental Disease,* Vol. 153, No. 5, (November 1971), pp. 351-359

Carter, C.S., Macdonald, A.M., Botvinick, M., Ross, L.L., Stenger, V.A., Noll, D. et al. (2000). Parsing executive processes: Strategic versus evaluative functions of the anterior cingulate cortex. *Proceedings of the National Academy of Sciences,* Vol. 97, No. 4, (February 15 2000), pp. 1944-1948

Carter, C.S., MacDonald III, A.W., Ross, L.L. & Stenger, V.A. (2001). Anterior cingulate cortex activity and impaired self-monitoring of performance in patients with schizophrenia: An event-related fMRI study. *American Journal of Psychiatry*, Vol. 158, No. 9, (September 2001), pp. 1423-1428

Dassonville, P., Lewis, S.M., Zhu, X-H., Ugurbil, K., Kim, S-G. & Ashe, J. (2001). The effect of stimulus-response compatibility on cortical motor activation. *Neuroimage*, Vol. 13, No. 1, (January 2001), pp. 1-14

Fan, J., Wu, Y., Fossella, J.A. & Posner, M.I. (2001). Assessing the heritability of attentional networks, *BMC Neuroscience*, Vol. 2, No. , (September 2001), pp. 2-14

Fan, J., McCandliss, B.D., Fossella, J., Flombaum, J.I. & Posner, M.I. (2005). The activation of attentional networks. *Neuroimage*, Vol. 26, No. 2, (June 2005), pp. 1471-479

Gallinat, J., Mulert, C., Bajbouj, M., Herrmann, W.M., Schunter, J., Senkowski, D. et al. (2002). Frontal and temporal dysfunction of auditory stimulus processing schizophrenia. *Neuroimage*, Vol. 17, No. 1, (September 2002), 110-127.

Green, M.F. (1996). What are the functional consequences of neurocognitive deficits in schizophrenia. *American Journal of Psychiatry*, Vol. 153, No. 3, (March 1996), pp. 321-330.

Green, M.F., Kern, R.S., Braff, D.L., & Mintz, J. (2000). Neurocognitive deficits and functional outcome in schizophrenia: Are we measuring the "Right Stuff"?. *Schizophrenia Bulletin*, Vol. 26, No. 1, (2000), pp. 119-136.

Hallmayer, J.F., Kalaydjieva, L., Badcock, J., Dragovic, M., Howell, S., Michie, P. et al. (2005). Genetic evidence for a distinct subtype of schizophrenia characterized by pervasive cognitive deficit. *American Journal of Human Genetics*, Vol. 77, No. 3, (September 2005), pp. 468-476.

Huston, P.E., Shakow, D., & Riggs, L.A. (1937). Studies of motor function in schizophrenia: II. Reaction time. *Journal of General Psychology*, Vol. 16, pp. 39-82 ISSN: 0022-1309

Iacoboni, M., Woods, R.P., & Mazziotta, J.C. (1996). Brain-behavior relationships: Evidence from practice effects in spatial stimulus-response compatibility. *Journal of Neurophysiology*, Vol. 76, No. 1, (July 1996), pp. 321-331

Jansma, J.M., Ramsey, N.F., Slagter, H.A. & Kahn, R.S. (2001). Functional anatomical correlates of controlled and automatic processing. *Journal of Cognitive Neuroscience*, Vol. 13, No. 6, (August 2001), pp. 730-743, ISSN: 0898-929X

Jiang, Y. & Kanwisher, N. (2003). Common neural substrates for response selection across modalities and mapping paradigms, *Journal of Cognitive Neuroscience*, Vol. 15, No. 8, (November 2003), pp. 1080-1094, ISSN: 0898-929X

Jiang, Y. & Kanwisher, N. (2003a). Common neural mechanisms for response selection and perceptual processing, *Journal of Cognitive Neuroscience*, Vol. 15, No. 8, (November 2003), pp. 1095-1110, ISSN: 0898-929X

Kiana, R., Shanks, T.D. & Shadlen, M.N. (2006). When is enough enough? *Nature Neuroscience*, Vol. 9, No. 7, (July 2006), pp. 861-863, ISSN: 1097-6256

Lo, C-C. & Wang, X-J. (2006). Cortico-basal ganglia circuit mechanism for a decision threshold in reaction time tasks. *Nature Neuroscience*, Vol. 9, No. 7, (July 2006), pp. 956- 963, ISSN: 1097-6256

Luciano, M., Wright, M.J., Geffen, G.M., Geffen, L.B., Smith, G.A. & Martin, N G. (2004). A genetic investigation of the covariation among inspection time, choice reaction time, and IQ subtest scores. *Behavior Genetics*, Vol. 34, No. 1, (January 2004), pp. 41-50.

Luck, S.J., Fuller, R.L., Braun, E.L., Robinson, B., Summerfelt, A. & Gold, J.M. (2006). The speed of visual attention in schizophrenia: Electrophysiological and behavioural evidence, *Schizophrenia Research*, Vol.85, No. 1-3, (July 2006), pp. 174-195

Luck, S.J., Kappenman, E.S., Fuller, R.L., Robinson, B., Summerfelt, A. & Gold, J.M. (2009). Impaired response selection in schizophrenia: Evidence from the P3 wave and the lateralized readiness potential, *Psychophysiology*, Vol.46, No. 4, (July 2009), pp. 776-786, ISSN: 1469-8986

MacDonald, III, A.W., Cohen, J.D., Stenger, V.A. & Carter, C.S. (2000). Dissociating the role of the dorsolaterla prefrontal and anterior cingulate cortex in cognitive control. *Science*, Vol. 288, No. 5472, (9 June 2000), pp. 1835-1838

Margulies, D.S., Kelly, A.M.C., Uddin, L.Q., Biswal, B.B., Castellanos, F.X., & Milham, M.P. (2007). Mapping the functional connectivity of anterior cingulate cortex. *NeuroImage*, Vol. 37, No. 2, (August 2007), pp. 579-588

Matza, L., Brewster, J., Revicki, D., Zhao, Y., Purdon, S.E. & Buchanan, R. (2006). Measuring changes in functional status among patients with schizophrenia: The link with cognitive impairment. *Schizophrenia Bulletin*, Vol. 32, No. 4, (October 2006), pp. 666-678

McAllindon, D.P., Wilman, A.H., Purdon, S.E., & Tibbo, P.G. (2010). Functional magnetic resonance imaging of choice reaction time in chronic schizophrenia and first-degree relatives. *Schizophrenia Research*, Vol. 120, No. 1-3, (July 2010), pp.232-233

Mulert, C., Gallinat, J., Pacual-Marqui, R., Dorn, H., Frick, K., Schlattmann, P. et al. (2001). Reduced event-related current density in the anterior cingulate cortex in schizophrenia. *Neuroimage*, Vol. 13, No. 4, (April 2001), pp. 589-600

Mulert, C., Gallinat, J., Dorn, H., Herrmann, W.M. & Winterer, G. (2003). The relationship between reaction time, error rate and anterior cingulate cortex activity. *International Journal of Psychophysiology*, Vol. 47, No. 2, (February 2003), pp. 175-183

Mulert, C., Menzinger, E., Leicht, G., Pogarell, O. & Hegerl, U. (2005). Evidence for a close relationship between conscious effort and anterior cingulate activity. *International Journal of Psychophysiology*, Vol. 56, No. 1, (April 2005), pp. 65-80.

Naito, E., Kinomura, S., Geyer, S., Kawashima, R., Roland, P.E. & Zilles, K., (2000). Fast reaction to different sensory modalities activates common fields in the motor areas, but the anterior cingulate cortex is involved in the speed of reaction. *Journal of Neurophysiology*, Vol. 83, No. 3, (March 2000), pp. 1701-1709.

Ngan, E.T.C. & Liddle, P.F., (2000). Reaction time, symptom profiles and course of illness in schizophrenia. *Schizophrenia Research*, Vol. 46, No. 2-3, (December 2000), pp. 195-201

Nuechterlein, K.H. (1977). Reaction time and attention in schizophrenia: A critical evaluation of the data and theories, *Schizophrenia Bulletin*, Vol. 3, No. 3, (1977), pp. 373-428

Ogawa, S., Lee, T.M., Kay, A.R. & Tank D.W. (1990). Brain Magnetic Resonance Imaging With Contrast Dependent on Blood Oxygenation. *Proceedings of the National Academies of Sciences USA*, Vol. 87, No. , pp. 9868-9872.

Pellizzer, G. & Stephane, M. (2007). Response selection in schizophrenia. *Experimental Brain Research*, Vol. 180, No. 4, (July 2007), pp. 705-714

Picard, N. & Strick, P.L. (1996). Motor areas of the medial wall: A review of their location and functional activation. *Cerebral Cortex*, Vol. 6, No. 3, (May 1996), pp. 342-353.

Posner, M.I. & DiGirolamo, G.J. (1998). Executive attention: conflict, target detection, and cognitive control. In: *The Attentive Brain*, R. Parasuraman Ed., pp.401-423, MIT Press, Cambridge, MA

Praamstra, P., Kourtis, D., Kwok,H.F. & Oostenveld, R. (2006). Neurophysiology of implicit timing in serial choice reaction-time performance. *The Journal of Neuroscience*, Vol. 26, No. 20, (17 May 2006), pp. 5448-5455, ISSN: 0270-6474

Rijsdijk, F.V., Vernon, P.A. & Boomsma, D.I. (1998). The genetic basis of the relation between speed-of-information-processing and IQ. *Behavioural Brain Research*, Vol. 95, No. 1, (September 1998), pp. 77-84.

Roitman, J.D. & Shadlen, M.N. (2002). Response of neurons in the lateral intraprietal area during a combined visual discrimination reaction time task. *The Journal of Neuroscience*, Vol. 22, No. 21, (1 November 2002), pp. 9475-9489, ISSN: 0270-6474

Schall, J.D. (2002). The neural selection and control of saccades by the frontal eye field. *Philosophical Transactions of the Royal Society of London B Biological Sciences*, Vol. 357, No. 1424, (August 2002), pp. 1073-1082

Schumacher, E.H. & Jiang, Y. (2003). Neural mechanisms for response selection: Representation specific or modality independent?, *Journal of Cognitive Neuroscience*, Vol. 15, No. 8, (November 2003), pp. 1077-1079, ISSN: 0898-929X

Schumacher, E.H., Elston, P.A. & D'Esposito, M. (2003). Neural evidence for representation-specific response selection, *Journal of Cognitive Neuroscience*, Vol. 15, No. 8, (November 2003), pp. 1111-1121, ISSN: 0898-929X

Silverstein, S.M., Schenkel, L.S., Valone, C. & Nuernberger, S.W. (1998). Cognitive deficits and psychiatric rehabilitation outcomes in schizophrenia. *Psychiatric Quarterly*, Vol. 69, No. 3, (September 1998), pp. 169-191.

Smith, P.L. & Ratcliff, R. (2004). Psychology and neurobiology of simple decisions. *Trends in Neurosciences,* Vol. 27, No. 3, (March 2004), pp. 161-168

Swick, D. & Jovanovic, J. (2002). Anterior cingulate cortex and the Stroop task: neuropsychological evidence for topographic specificity. *Neuropsychologia,* Vol. 40, No. 8, (2002), pp. 1240-1253

Taylor, S.F., Kornblum, S., Minoshima, S., Oliver, L.M. & Koeppe, R.A. (1994). Changes in medial cortical blood flow with a stimulus-response compatibility task. *Neuropsychologia,* Vol. 32, No. 2, (February 1994), pp. 249-255

Thoma, R.J., Yeo, R.A., Gangestad, S., Halgren, E., Davis, J., Paulson, K.M. & Lewine, J.D. (2006). Developmental instability and the neural dynamics of the speed-intelligence relationship, *NeuroImage,* Vol. 32, No. 3,(September 2006), pp. 1456-1464

Tuch,D.S., Salat,D.H., Wisco,J.J., Zaleta,A.K., Hevelone,N.D. and Rosas,H.D. (2005). Choice reaction time performance correlates with diffusion anisotropy in white matter pathways supporting visuospatial attention. *Proceedings of the National Academy of Sciences U S A.,* Vol. 102, No. 34, (August 23 2005), pp. 12212-12217.

Vogt, B.A., Finch, D.M. & Olson, C.R. (1992). Functional heterogeneity in cingulate cortex: The anterior executive and posterior evaluative regions. *Cerebral Cortex,* Vol. 2, No. 6, (November 1992), pp. 435-443.

Wells & Kelley, (1922). The simple reaction time in psychosis. *American Journal of Psychiatry,* Vol. 79, No. 1, (July 1922), pp. 53-59.

Winterer, G., Mulert, C., Mientus, S., Gallinat, J., Schlattmann, P., Dorn, H. et al. (2001). P300 and LORETA: Comparison of normal subjects and schizophrenic patients. *Brain Topography,* Vol. 13, No. 4, (June 2001), pp. 299-313.

Winterer, G., Adams, C.M., Jones, D.W. & Knutson, B. (2002). Volition to action - An event-related fMRI study. *Neuroimage,* Vol. 17, No. 2, (October 2002), pp. 851-858.

Wong, K-F. & Wang, X-J. (2006). A recurrent network mechanism of time integration in perceptual decision. *Journal of Neuroscience,* Vol. 26, No. 4, (25 January 2006), pp. 1314-1328.

Woodward N.D., Tibbo, P.G. & Purdon SE (2007). An fMRI investigation of procedural learning in unaffected siblings of individuals with schizophrenia. *Schizophrenia Research,* Vol. 94, No. 1-3, (August 2007), pp. 306-316.

Woodward, N.D., Waldie, B., Rogers, B., Tibbo, P., Seres, P. & Purdon, S.E. (2009). Abnormal prefrontal cortical activity and connectivity during response selection in first episode psychosis, chronic schizophrenia, and unaffected siblings of individuals with schizophrenia, *Schizophrenia Research,* Vol. 109, No. 1-3, (April 2009), pp. 182-190

Wright, M., De Geus, E., Ando, J., Luciano, M., Posthuma, D., Ono, Y. et al. (2001). Genetics of cognition: Outline of a collaborative twin study. *Twin Research and Human Genetics,* Vol. 4, No. 1, (2001), pp. 48-56, ISSN: 1832-4274

Yarkoni, T., Barch, D.M., Gray, J.R., Conturo, T.E. & Braver, T.S (2009). BOLD correlates of trial-by-trial reaction time variability in gray and white matter: A multi-study fMRI analysis, *PLoS ONE,* Vol. 4, No. 1, (January 2009), pp. 1-15

Zahn, T.P., & Carpenter, W.T., (1978). Effects of short term outcome and clinical improvement on RT in acute schizophrenia. *Journal of Psychiatric Research,* Vol. 14, pp. 59-68.

Zedkova, L., Woodward, N.D., Harding, I., Tibbo, P.G. & Purdon, S.E. (2006). Procedural learning in schizophrenia investigated with functional magnetic resonance imaging. *Schizophrenia Research*, Vol. 88, No. 1-3, (December 2006), pp. 198-207.

Part 3

Preclinical Research on Schizophrenia

7

Serotonin-1A Receptors and Cognitive Enhancement in Schizophrenia: Role for Brain Energy Metabolism

Tomiki Sumiyoshi and Takashi Uehara
Department of Neuropsychiatry, Graduate School of Medicine and Pharmaceutical Sciences, University of Toyama
Japan

1. Introduction

Disturbances of cognitive function, evaluated by psychological and neurophysiological methods, have been shown to predict outcome in patients with schizophrenia (Green et al. 2000, Javitt et al. 2008, Sumiyoshi T. et al. 2011). In view of the paucity of treatment options to improve cognition for these patients, efforts to identify novel strategies are needed.

The prefrontal cortex (PFC) has been considered to regulate various aspects of cognitive abilities, e.g. working memory, memory organization, executive function, and attention (Sumiyoshi T. et al. 2011). Atypical antipsychotic drugs (AAPDs), eliciting cognitive benefits to some extent, enhance dopamine (DA) release in the medial PFC (mPFC), as demonstrated by in vivo microdialysis (Bortolozzi et al. 2010, Diaz-Mataix et al. 2005, Ichikawa et al. 2001). The ability of AAPDs to enhance DA in mPFC has been found to depend on serotonin (5-HT)-5-HT_{1A} receptors, irrespective of direct in vitro affinity, based on observations from mutant mice lacking these receptors (Bortolozzi et al. 2010, Diaz-Mataix et al. 2005). This is consistent with behavioral observations that 5-HT_{1A} partial agonists (e.g. tandospirone) and AAPDs with agonist actions on 5-HT_{1A} receptors (e.g. perospirone, aripiprazole, ziprasidone, lurasidone) ameliorate memory deficits in rodent models of schizophrenia (Hagiwara et al. 2008, Horiguchi et al. in press, Meltzer et al. 2011, Nagai et al. 2009). Findings from electrophysiological studies suggest these cognitive benefits of 5-HT_{1A} agonism are mediated by glutamate (Glu) and γ-aminobutyric acid (GABA) neurons (Higuchi et al. 2010, Llado-Pelfort et al. 2011).

In this chapter, the authors discuss the role for the key 5-HT receptor subtypes, i.e., 5-HT_{1A}, 5-HT_{2A}, 5-HT_6, and 5-HT_7 receptors, in cognitive function in schizophrenia. Specifically, we will focus on several psychotropic/antipsychotic compounds stimulating 5-HT_{1A} receptors, considered as one of the most promising candidates for cognitive enhancers (Meltzer et al. 2011, Newman-Tancredi and Kleven 2011, Newman-Tancredi and Albert in press). A hypothesis is presented on the relationship between cognition and lactate that provides an important energy substrate and reflects neural activity in the brain.

2. Neurocognitive deficits of schizophrenia

Schizophrenia has been characterized by positive symptoms (e.g. delusions, hallucinations and thought disorder) and negative symptoms (e.g. psychomotor retardation, affective flattening, social withdrawal, and alogia). Patients with the illness also exhibit a wide range of disturbances of cognitive function, including several types of memory, executive function (e.g. planning, monitoring, inhibition), vigilance, motor speed, and verbal fluency, with more than 1SD below the average of normal controls (Harvey and Keefe 1997).

Generally, they are considered to be independent of the psychotic symptoms. The cognitive deficits of schizophrenia have been investigated extensively as a determinant of functional outcome (Addington and Addington 2000, Green 1996, Green et al. 2000).

Several instruments to comprehensively assess cognitive function in schizophrenia have been developed. In particular, the Measurement and Treatment Research to Improve Cognition in Schizophrenia (MATRICS) Consensus Cognitive Battery (Nuechterlein et al. 2008) (Fig 1) and the Brief Assessment of Cognition in Schizophrenia (BACS) (Keefe et al. 2004) (Fig 2) are regarded to be qualified as international-standard neuropsychological tools in this respect. The authors have developed the Japanese versions of these cognitive test batteries (Kaneda et al. 2007, Sato et al. 2010), and have confirmed their sensitivity and validity to detect cognitive deficits in patients (Fig 3).

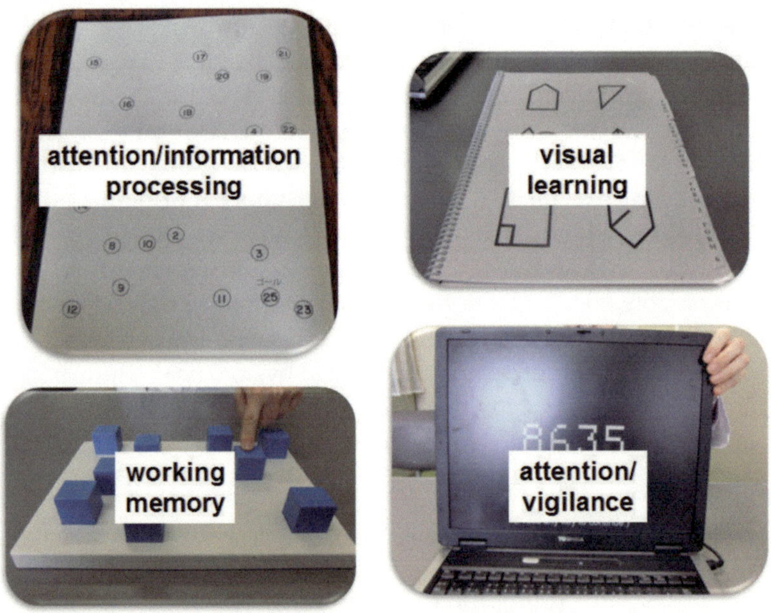

Fig. 1. Examples of tests from the MATRICS Consensus Cognitive Battery.

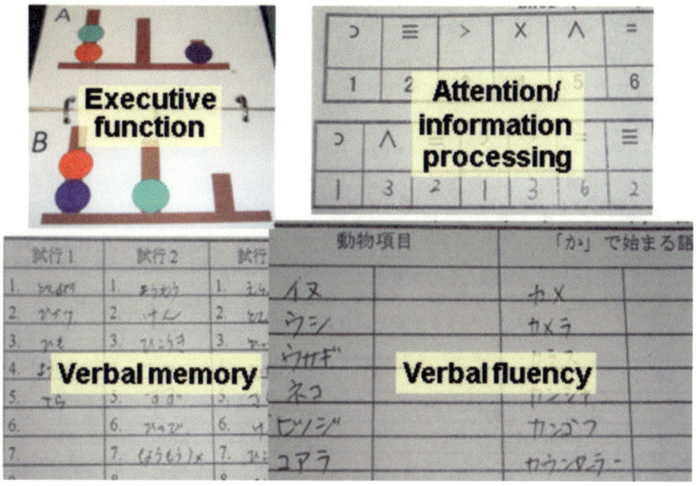

Fig. 2. Examples of tests from the Brief Assessment of Cognition in Schizophrenia.

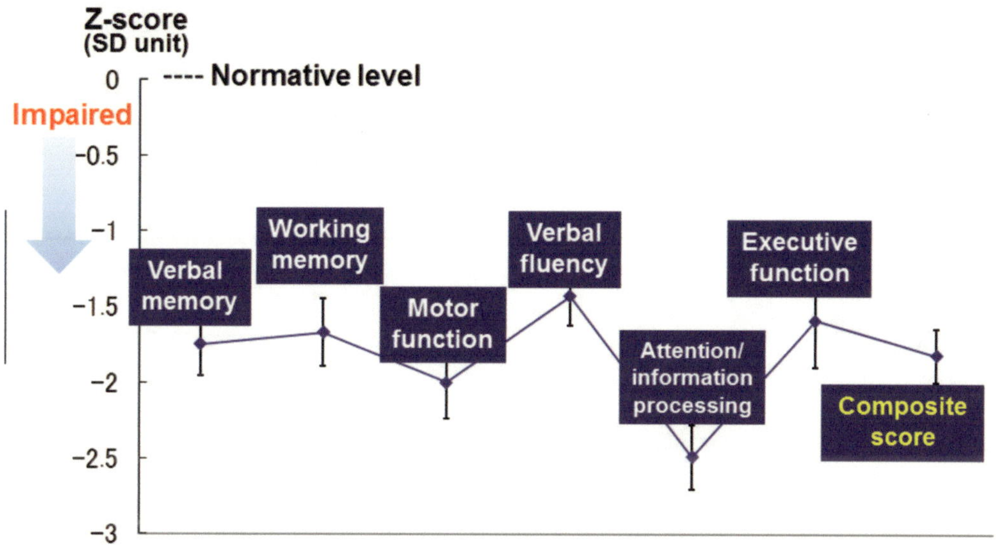

Fig. 3. Impaired cognitive function in schizophrenia as evaluated by the Brief Assessment of Cognition in Schizophrenia -Japanese Version (Kaneda et al. 2007).

3. 5-HT receptors and cognitive function

The role for several subtypes of 5-HT receptors in cognitive function has attracted interest, based, partly, on the distinct pharmacological properties of AAPDs, such as clozapine, risperidone, and olanzapine. For example, the ability of these agents to enhance DA and acetylcholine release in the mPFC, demonstrated by in vivo microdialysis, has been reported (Bortolozzi et al. 2010, Diaz-Mataix et al. 2005, Ichikawa et al. 2002, Ichikawa et al. 2001). Among the subtypes of 5-HT receptors (Fig. 4), 5-HT$_{1A}$, 5-HT$_{2A}$, 5-HT$_6$, and 5-HT$_7$ receptors have been shown to be associated with cognitive effects of AAPDs, suggesting pivotal roles for the serotonergic system in cognitive symptoms of schizophrenia (Sumiyoshi T. et al. 2007a, Meltzer and Sumiyoshi 2008, Sumiyoshi T. et al. 2008).

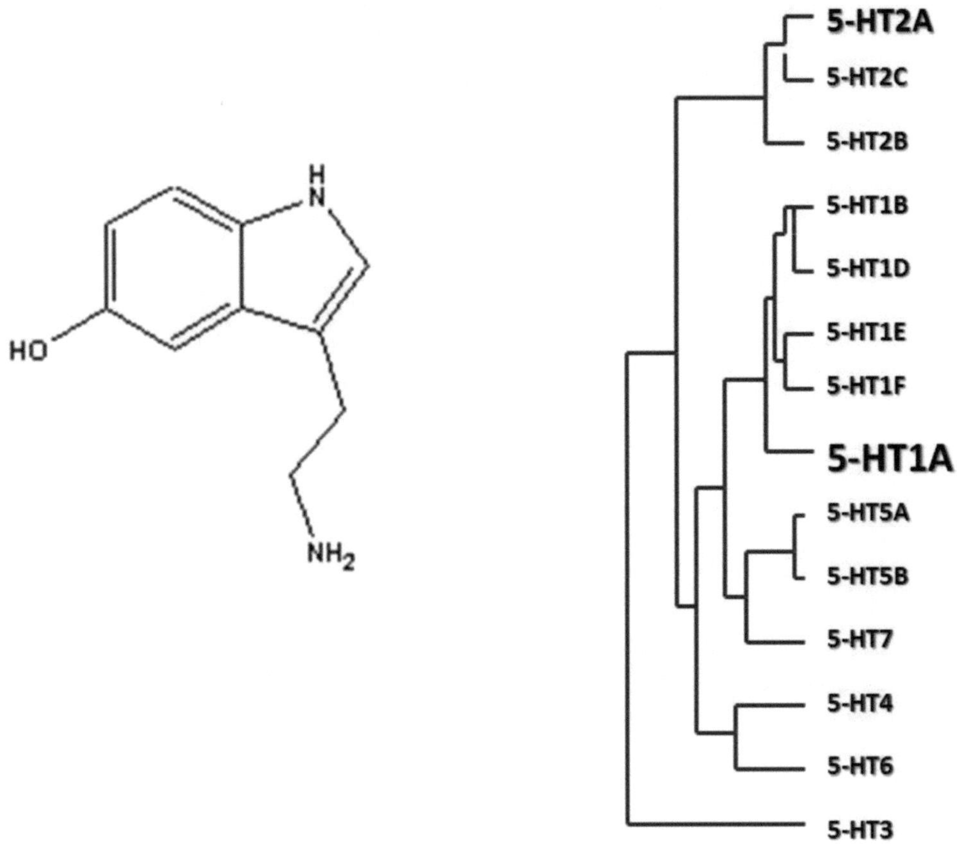

Fig. 4. Chemical structure of serotonin (5-HT) and its receptor subtypes.

Table 1. summarizes the mode of actions (agonism or antagonism) and specific compounds related to the above-mentioned 5-HT receptor subtypes. Among them, 5-HT_{1A} receptor stimulation is currently considered as the most promising approach (Llado-Pelfort et al. 2011, Newman-Tancredi and Kleven 2011, Newman-Tancredi and Albert in press, Sumiyoshi C. et al. 2006, Sumiyoshi T. et al. 2008, Sumiyoshi T. et al. 2007a, Sumiyoshi T. et al. 2000, Sumiyoshi T. et al. 2007b, Sumiyoshi T. et al. 2001a, Sumiyoshi T. et al. 2001b, Sumiyoshi T. et al. 2009), as discussed in the next section. This is followed by 5-HT_{2A} antagonism, as elicited by certain (although not satisfactory) efficacy of a series of AAPDs whose principal pharmacologic feature is blockade of 5-HT_{2A} receptors (Meltzer et al. 1989, Meltzer et al. 2011, Meltzer and Massey 2011, Stockmeier et al. 1993, Sumiyoshi T. et al. 1995). Recent evidence from animal models of schizophrenia suggests the advantage of agonists at 5-HT_6 or 5-HT_7 receptors for ameliorating memory impairment, as revealed by behavioral experiments using antagonist at the N-methyl-D-aspartate (NMDA) type of Glu receptors (Horiguchi et al. 2011, Meltzer et al. 2011, Meltzer and Massey 2011).

5-HT subtypes	Mode of actions	Compounds
$5\text{-}HT_{1A}$	(partial) agonist	tandospirone, buspirone F15599, ziprasidone aripiprazole, perospirone lurasidone
$5\text{-}HT_{2A}$	antagonist	clozapine, risperidone olanzapine, perospirone quetiapine, melperone N-desmethylclozapine
$5\text{-}HT_6$	antagonist	Ro04-6790 Lu AE58054
$5\text{-}HT_7$	antagonist	SB25874 amisulpiride lurasidone

Ref) Harvey et al. 2011; Kern et al. 2006; Llado-Pelfort et al. 2010, 2011; Meltzer et al. 2011; Meltzer and Massey 2011; Newman-Tancredi 2011, in press; Sumiyoshi et al. 2000, 2001a, 2001b, 2006, 2007a, 2007b, 2008, 2009

Table 1. Serotonin (5-HT) receptors in the treatment of cognitive disturbances.

4. Role for $5\text{-}HT_{1A}$ stimulation in cognitive enhancement

The interest in the $5\text{-}HT_{1A}$ receptor in relation to cognition in schizophrenia was founded by a series of pilot studies of the effects of augmentation therapy with tandospirone, a $5\text{-}HT_{1A}$ partial agonist, in patients treated with antipsychotic drugs (Sumiyoshi T. et al. 2000, Sumiyoshi T. et al. 2001a, Sumiyoshi T. et al. 2001b). The addition of tandospirone (30 mg/day), but not placebo, to typical antipsychotic drugs (mainly haloperidol) for 4–6 weeks, was found to improve verbal memory (effect size = 0.70), memory organization, and executive function (0.63) (Sumiyoshi T. et al. 2000, Sumiyoshi T. et al. 2001a, Sumiyoshi T. et al. 2001b).

The beneficial effect of augmentation therapy with $5\text{-}HT_{1A}$ agonists in schizophrenia was further supported by a randomly assigned placebo-controlled double-blind study with buspirone, another $5\text{-}HT_{1A}$ partial agonist (Sumiyoshi T. et al. 2007a). Patients with schizophrenia, who had been treated with an atypical antipsychotic drug, were assigned to receive either buspirone, 30 mg/day, or matching placebo for 6 months. Buspirone outperformed placebo in improving the performance on a measure of attention/speeded motor performance (effect size = 0.32), indicating an advantage for cognitive abilities regulated by prefrontal cortex, as in the case of tandospirone. Evidence from these proof-of-concept studies has prompted the recent endeavor to develop cognition-enhancing drugs with $5\text{-}HT_{1A}$ agonist actions (Depoortere et al. 2010, Llado-Pelfort et al. 2010, Llado-Pelfort et al. 2011, Newman-Tancredi 2010, Newman-Tancredi and Kleven 2011, Newman-Tancredi and Albert in press). Some of the compounds so far synthesized in this line are shown in Fig 5.

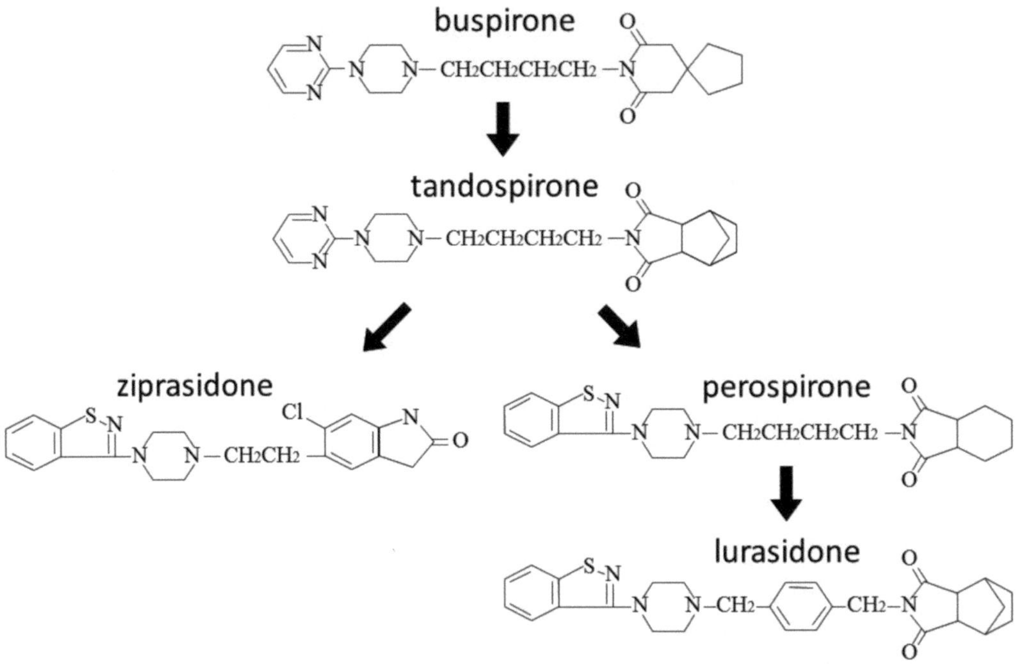

Fig. 5. Some of the psychotropic/antipsychotic compounds with agonist actions on 5-HT_{1A} receptors.

Support for this therapeutic strategy comes from animal data suggesting 5-HT_{1A} partial agonists (e.g. tandospirone) and AAPDs with agonist actions on 5-HT_{1A} receptors (e.g. perospirone, aripiprazole, ziprasidone, lurasidone) ameliorate memory deficits due to NMDA receptor blockade (Hagiwara et al. 2008, Horiguchi et al. 2011, Horiguchi et al. in press, Meltzer et al. 2011, Nagai et al. 2009). The ability of these compounds to improve cognition has been related to enhancement of extracellular concentration of DA in the PFC (Bortolozzi et al. 2010, Diaz-Mataix et al. 2005, Ichikawa et al. 2001, Yoshino et al. 2004), an effect which is absent in mutant mice lacking 5-HT_{1A} (Bortolozzi et al. 2010, Diaz-Mataix et al. 2005), but not 5-HT_{2A} (Bortolozzi et al. 2010) receptors.

As illustrated in Fig. 6, Glu, GABA, 5-HT, and DA neurons constitute a network in the PFC that regulates several domains of cognition, e.g. some types of memory, executive function and attention. Among the variety of relevant receptors in this neural cascade, 5-HT_{1A} receptors are located on Glu (pyramidal) and GABA neurons. Excitation of pyramidal neurons projecting to ventral tegmental area enhances mesocortical DA function, leading to amelioration of negative and cognitive symptoms of schizophrenia (Llado-Pelfort et al. 2010, Llado-Pelfort et al. 2011). Specifically, systemic administration of 8-OH-DPAT, a prototypical 5-HT_{1A} agonist, to rats increased the discharge rate of pyramidal neurons in mPFC, by inhibiting fast-spiking GABAergic interneurons through a preferential action on 5-HT_{1A} receptors on these latter neurons (Llado-Pelfort et al. 2011). This finding reconciles the observations that endogenous 5-HT inhibits pyramidal neurons in mPFC, while systemic administration of 5-HT_{1A} agonists excites them. These considerations are consistent with the clinical observation that augmentation therapy with tandospirone enhanced mismatch negativity, an electrophysiological cognitive marker of Glu neuron activity, in schizophrenia (Higuchi et al. 2010).

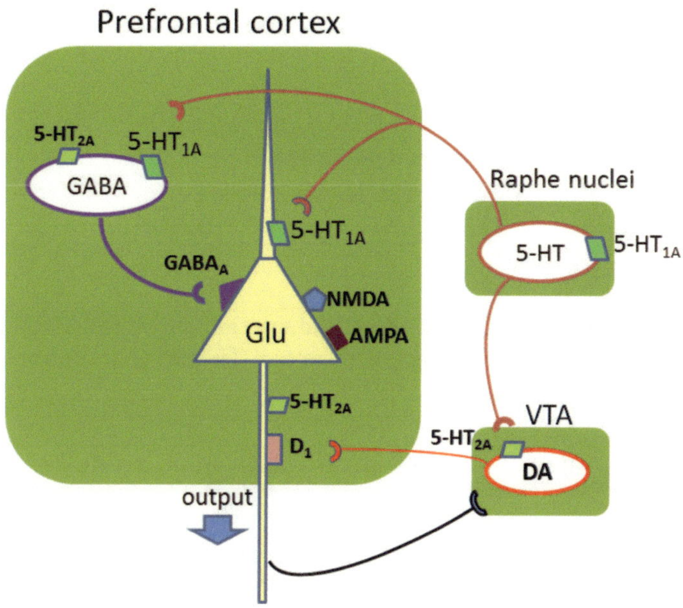

Fig. 6. Neural network in the prefrontal cortex involving glutamate, GABA, 5-HT and DA neurons. Part of the effect of 5-HT_{1A} agonists on cognition and negative symptoms is thought to be mediated by 5-HT_{1A} receptors located on GABAergic interneurons regulating glutamatergic pyramidal neurons. VTA, ventral tegmental area.

5. Lactate in brain energy metabolism

Although glucose has been considered to be a major supplier of energy in the brain, recent investigations report that lactate also plays a significant role in energy metabolism, especially during acute neural activation (Aubert et al. 2005, O'Brien et al. 2007). According to the "astrocyte-neuron lactate shuttle hypothesis" (Laughton et al. 2007, Pellerin 2003), lactate is produced in a neural activity-dependent and glutamate-mediated manner by astrocytes, and is transferred to and used by active neurons (reviewed in Uehara et al. 2008) (Fig. 7). Data from a recent study (Wyss et al. 2011) suggest that the brain prefers lactate over glucose as an energy substrate when both are available, and that lactate exerts a direct neuroprotective effect.

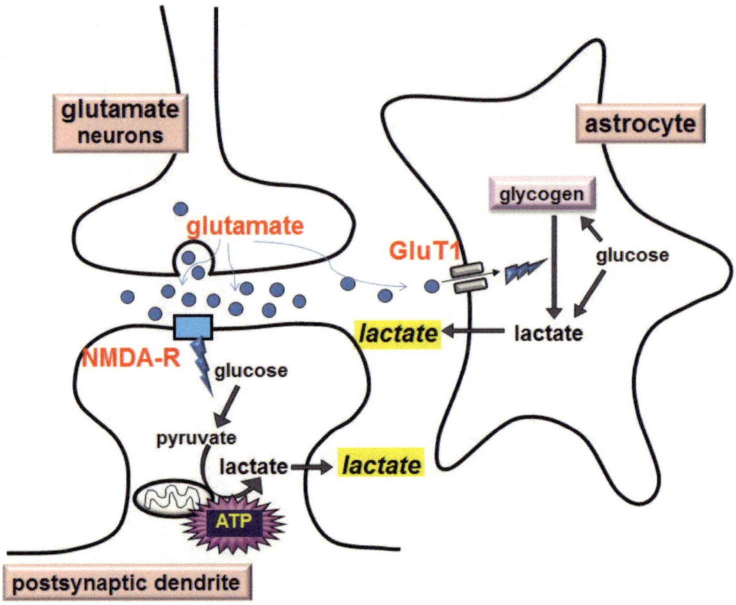

Fig. 7. Enhancement of lactate production by glutamatergic transmission. GluT1, glutamate transporter; NMDA-R, N-methyl-D-aspartate receptor. (Uehara et al. *Pharmacol Biochem Behav* 90:273, 2008)

6. Role for 5-HT_{1A} agonism in lactate production in an animal model of schizophrenia

Rats administered MK-801 on postnatal days (PD) 7-10 have been shown to elicit impairment of set-shifting test, a measure of prefrontal cortex function, in early adulthood (Stefani and Moghaddam 2005). The same model animals elicit disruption of prepulse inhibition, a measure of sensorimotor gating (Uehara et al. 2009, Uehara et al. 2010) and enhancement of spontaneous and metamphetamine-induced locomotor activity (Uehara et al. 2010) after, but not before puberty (Table 2). These findings suggest that transient blockade of NMDA receptors at the neonatal stage produces cognitive abnormalities in rodent models of schizophrenia based on the neurodevelopmental hypothesis of the illness.

Lactate metabolism in mPFC has been shown to be modulated by 5-HT_{1A} receptors both during resting condition and acute neural activation. In particular, acute administration of tandospirone led to a significant increase in extracellular lactate concentrations, and reduced the footshock stress-induced lactate increment in the mPFC in rats (Uehara et al. 2006). Taken together, it was hypothesized that transient blockade of NMDA receptors during the neonatal stage (modeling schizophrenia) would inhibit energy demands in response to stress in the mPFC at the young adult stage, and that 5-HT_{1A} partial agonist, such as tandospirone, would reverse the effect of the neonatal insult on energy metabolism.

Female Wistar rats obtained at 14 days of pregnancy. At postnatal (PD) day 7 (PD7), male pups were randomly divided into two groups. They received MK-801 (dizocilpine), or an equal volume of saline (control; vehicle group) once daily for 4 days. At the time of weaning on PD 21, the pups were grouped into four to six per treatment.

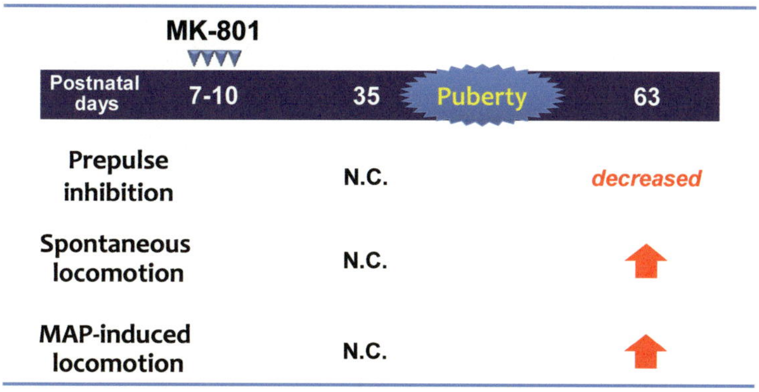

Transient blockade of NMDA receptors by MK-801 at the neonatal stage produces disruption of prepulse inhibition, as well as spontaneous or methamphetamine (MAP)-induced hyperlocomotion after, but not before puberty.
N.C., no change.

Table 2. Behavioral changes in a rat model of schizophrenia based on the neurodevelopmental hypothesis.

On PD49, animals were assigned to receive either saline or tandospirone at 1.0 mg/kg, (s.c.). This yielded the following groups: saline-saline group, saline-tandospirone group, MK801-saline group, and MK801-tandospirone group. For 14 days before the microdialysis examination, saline or tandospirone was administered (s.c.) once daily. Microdialysis was performed 24 hours after the last injection.

Microdialysis experiments were performed on PD63. Forty-two to 48 hr before microdialysis experiments, the animals were anesthetized, and were mounted on a stereotaxic apparatus. A dialysis probe was implanted into the left mPFC with the coordinates of A 3.2mm, L 0.6mm, V 5.2mm from bregma. The dialysis experiment was carried out on the freely moving rats. Artificial CSF was perfused into the dialysis probe. The dialysates were mixed on-line with an enzyme solution containing L-lactate dehydrogenate and NAD+ in a T-tube. During transport of the mixture to the fluorometer, lactate was enzymatically oxidized and the fluorescence of the nicotinamid adenosine dinucleotide diphosphate (NADH) formed was continuously measured, with a standard solution of 100 µmol/L lactate for calibration.

Footshock stress was administered using a plastic communication box, according to the method described previously (Uehara et al., 2006). The box (L 51cm x W 51cm x H 40cm) was equipped with a grid floor, and was subdivided into nine compartments (17cm x17cm) by transparent plastic walls. In this study, we used 4 compartments area (34cm x 34cm) for the field of free moving and footshock administration. The communication box was connected to a shock-generator to deliver footshocks as described below. Each footshock session consisted of a scramble shock of 0.3 mA for 5 seconds administered every 30 seconds for 10 minutes. After the experimental sessions, the position of dialysis probes was verified by dissection of the brain.

Data were analyzed by analysis of variance (ANOVA). The average of extracellular lactate concentrations during the period preceding the start of footshock stress (ten measurements performed every 2 min) was used as the control value (100 %). Data from tandospirone administration experiments were analyzed using three-way repeated measures ANOVA; Status and Drug were treated as between-group variables. Time was treated as a repeated measures variable.

As expected, transient neonatal administration of MK-801 suppressed lactate increment in response to footshock stress around puberty, which was reversed by 14-day treatment with tandospirone (Fig. 8). Further, the ability of tandospirone to ameliorate the response of lactate production in model animals was abolished by co-administration of WAY-100635, a selective 5-HT_{1A} antagonist (Uehara et al., in press).

These findings are consistent with clinical observations that perospirone and tandospirone improved cognitive abilities governed by the PFC, coupled with enhancement of electrophysiological activities in this brain region, in patients with schizophrenia (Higuchi et al. 2010, Sumiyoshi T. et al. 2009). Translational approach, like this, is expected to provide a novel insight into the development of therapeutics targeting cognitive disturbances of schizophrenia.

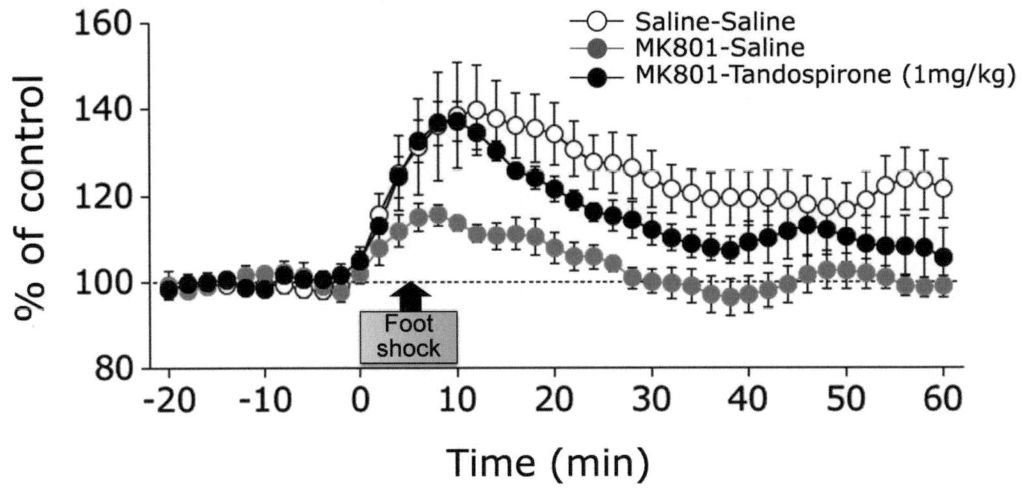

Fig. 8. Extracellular concentrations of lactate in the medial prefrontal cortex in young adult rats. Transient blockade of NMDA receptors by MK-801 at the neonatal stage (modeling schizophrenia) suppresses lactate increment in response to footshock stress (saline-saline vs. MK-801-saline). Treatment with tandospirone, a 5-HT_{1A} partial agonist, for 14 days reverses the decrease in lactate production in the model animals (MK-801-saline vs. MK801-tandospirone. A significant main effect of tandospirone in MK-801-treated animals was noted ($F(1,8)=12.94$, $P=0.007$ by ANOVA).

7. Conclusions

Behavioral, neurochemical and electrophysiological data indicate 5-HT_{1A} agonists improve negative symptoms and cognitive deficits of schizophrenia. Specifically, compelling evidence suggests that the cognitive benefits of 5-HT_{1A} agonism are mediated by Glu and

GABA neurons (Higuchi et al. 2010, Llado-Pelfort et al. 2011). The role for 5-HT_{1A} receptors in cognitive enhancement has been suggested by imaging genetics data regarding brain energy metabolism (Sumiyoshi T. et al. 2008) and by pharmacogenetics investigations (Sumiyoshi T. et al. 2010) [reviewed in (Newman-Tancredi and Kleven 2011, Newman-Tancredi and Albert in press)]. Findings from translational research, herein presented, are expected to facilitate the development of novel therapeutics for cognitive impairment in schizophrenia and other psychiatric disorders.

8. Acknowledgement

This work was supported by Health and Labour Sciences Research Grants and grants from Japan Society for Promotion of Sciences.

9. References

Addington J, Addington D. 2000. Neurocognitive and social functioning in schizophrenia: a 2.5 year follow-up study. Schizophr Res 44: 47-56.

Aubert A, Costalat R, Magistretti PJ, Pellerin L. 2005. Brain lactate kinetics: Modeling evidence for neuronal lactate uptake upon activation. Proc Natl Acad Sci U S A 102: 16448-16453.

Bortolozzi A, Masana M, Diaz-Mataix L, Cortes R, Scorza MC, Gingrich JA, Toth M, Artigas F. 2010. Dopamine release induced by atypical antipsychotics in prefrontal cortex requires 5-HT(1A) receptors but not 5-HT(2A) receptors. Int J Neuropsychopharmacol 13: 1299-1314.

Depoortere R, Auclair AL, Bardin L, Colpaert FC, Vacher B, Newman-Tancredi A. 2010. F15599, a preferential post-synaptic 5-HT1A receptor agonist: activity in models of cognition in comparison with reference 5-HT1A receptor agonists. Eur Neuropsychopharmacol 20: 641-654.

Diaz-Mataix L, Scorza MC, Bortolozzi A, Toth M, Celada P, Artigas F. 2005. Involvement of 5-HT1A receptors in prefrontal cortex in the modulation of dopaminergic activity: role in atypical antipsychotic action. J Neurosci 25: 10831-10843.

Green MF. 1996. What are the functional consequences of neurocognitive deficits in schizophrenia? . Am J Psychiatry 153: 321-330.

Green MF, Kern RS, Braff DL, Mintz J. 2000. Neurocognitive deficits and functional outcome in schizophrenia: Are we measuring the "right stuff"? Schizophr. Bull. 26: 119-136.

Hagiwara H, Fujita Y, Ishima T, Kunitachi S, Shirayama Y, Iyo M, Hashimoto K. 2008. Phencyclidine-induced cognitive deficits in mice are improved by subsequent subchronic administration of the antipsychotic drug perospirone: role of serotonin 5-HT1A receptors. Eur Neuropsychopharmacol 18: 448-454.

Harvey PD, Keefe RS. 1997. Cognitive impairment in schizophrenia and implication of atypical neuroleptic treatment. CNS spectrums 2: 41-55.

Higuchi Y, Sumiyoshi T, Kawasaki Y, Ito T, Seo T, Suzuki M. 2010. Effect of tandospirone on mismatch negativity and cognitive performance in schizophrenia: a case report. J Clin Psychopharmacol 30: 732-734.

Horiguchi M, Huang M, Meltzer HY. 2011. The role of 5-hydroxytryptamine 7 receptors in the phencyclidine-induced novel object recognition deficit in rats. J Pharmacol Exp Ther 338: 605-614.

Horiguchi M, Meltzer HY. in press. The role of $5\text{-}HT_{1A}$ receptors in phencyclidine-induced novel object recognition deficit in rats. Psychopharmacology.

Ichikawa J, Dai J, O'Laughlin IA, Fowler WL, Meltzer HY. 2002. Atypical, but not typical, antipsychotic drugs increase cortical acetylcholine release without an effect in the nucleus accumbens or striatum. Neuropsychopharmacology 26: 325-339.

Ichikawa J, Ishii H, Bonaccorso S, Fowler WL, O'Laughlin IA, Meltzer HY. 2001. 5-HT(2A) and D(2) receptor blockade increases cortical DA release via 5- HT(1A) receptor activation: a possible mechanism of atypical antipsychotic-induced cortical dopamine release. J Neurochem 76: 1521-1531.

Javitt DC, Spencer KM, Thaker GK, Winterer G, Hajos M. 2008. Neurophysiological biomarkers for drug development in schizophrenia. Nat Rev Drug Discov 7: 68-83.

Kaneda Y, Sumiyoshi T, Keefe R, Ishimoto Y, Numata S, Ohmori T. 2007. Brief assessment of cognition in schizophrenia: validation of the Japanese version. Psychiatry Clin Neurosci 61: 602-609.

Keefe RS, Goldberg TE, Harvey PD, Gold JM, Poe MP, Coughenour L. 2004. The Brief Assessment of Cognition in Schizophrenia: reliability, sensitivity, and comparison with a standard neurocognitive battery. Schizophr Res 68: 283-297.

Laughton JD, Bittar P, Charnay Y, Pellerin L, Kovari E, Magistretti PJ, Bouras C. 2007. Metabolic compartmentalization in the human cortex and hippocampus: evidence for a cell- and region-specific localization of lactate dehydrogenase 5 and pyruvate dehydrogenase. BMC Neurosci 8: 35.

Llado-Pelfort L, Assie MB, Newman-Tancredi A, Artigas F, Celada P. 2010. Preferential in vivo action of F15599, a novel 5-HT(1A) receptor agonist, at postsynaptic 5-HT(1A) receptors. Br J Pharmacol 160: 1929-1940.

Llado-Pelfort L, Santana N, Ghisi V, Artigas F, Celada P. 2011. 5-HT1A Receptor Agonists Enhance Pyramidal Cell Firing in Prefrontal Cortex Through a Preferential Action on GABA Interneurons. Cereb Cortex.

Meltzer HY, Sumiyoshi T. 2008. Does stimulation of 5-HT(1A) receptors improve cognition in schizophrenia? Behav Brain Res 195: 98-102.

Meltzer HY, Matsubara S, Lee JC. 1989. Classification of typical and atypical antipsychotic drugs on the basis of dopamine D-1, D-2 and serotonin2 pKi values. J Pharmacol Exp Ther 251: 238-246.

Meltzer HY, Horiguchi M, Massey BW. 2011. The role of serotonin in the NMDA receptor antagonist models of psychosis and cognitive impairment. Psychopharmacology (Berl) 213: 289-305.

Meltzer HY, Massey BW. 2011The role of serotonin receptors in the action of atypical antipsychotic drugs. Curr Opin Pharmacol 11:59-67.

Nagai T, Murai R, Matsui K, Kamei H, Noda Y, Furukawa H, Nabeshima T. 2009. Aripiprazole ameliorates phencyclidine-induced impairment of recognition memory through dopamine D1 and serotonin 5-HT1A receptors. Psychopharmacology (Berl) 202: 315-328.

Newman-Tancredi A. 2010. The importantce of $5\text{-}HT_{1A}$ receptor agonism in antipsychotic drug action: Rationale and perspectives. Curr Opin Investig Drugs 11: 802-812.

Newman-Tancredi A, Kleven MS. 2011. Comparative pharmacology of antipsychotics possessing combined dopamine D2 and serotonin 5-HT1A receptor properties. Psychopharmacology (Berl) 216: 451-473.

Newman-Tancredi A, Albert PR. in press. Gene polymorphism at serotonin 5-HT1A receptors; moving towards personalized medicine for psychosis and mood deficits? in Sumiyoshi T, ed. Schizophrenia Research: Recent Advances. New York: Nove Science Publishers.

Nuechterlein KH, et al. 2008. The MATRICS Consensus Cognitive Battery, part 1: test selection, reliability, and validity. Am J Psychiatry 165: 203-213.

O'Brien J, Kla KM, Hopkins IB, Malecki EA, McKenna MC. 2007. Kinetic parameters and lactate dehydrogenase isozyme activities support possible lactate utilization by neurons. Neurochem Res 32: 597-607.

Pellerin L. 2003. Lactate as a pivotal element in neuron-glia metabolic cooperation. Neurochem Int 43: 331-338.

Sato T, Kaneda Y, Sumiyoshi C, Sumiyoshi T, Sora I. 2010. Development of MATRICS Concensus Cognitive Battery- Japanese version; towards facilitation of schizophrenia therapeutics. Rinsho Seishin-yakuri (Clinical Psychopharmacology) 13:289-296 (in Japanese).

Stefani MR, Moghaddam B. 2005. Transient N-methyl-D-aspartate receptor blockade in early development causes lasting cognitive deficits relevant to schizophrenia. Biol Psychiatry 57: 433-436.

Stockmeier CA, DiCarlo JJ, Zhang Y, Thompson P, Meltzer HY. 1993. Characterization of typical and atypical antipsychotic drugs based on in vivo occupancy of $serotonin_2$ and $dopamine_2$ receptors. J. Pharmacol. Exp. Ther. 266: 1374-1384.

Sumiyoshi C, Sumiyoshi T, Roy A, Jayathilake K, Meltzer HY. 2006. Atypical antipsychotic drugs and organization of long-term semantic memory: multidimensional scaling and cluster analyses of category fluency performance in schizophrenia. Int J Neuropsychopharmacol 9: 677-683.

Sumiyoshi T, Bubenikova-Valesova V, Horacek J, Bert B. 2008. Serotonin1A receptors in the pathophysiology of schizophrenia: development of novel cognition-enhancing therapeutics. Adv Ther 25: 1037-1056.

Sumiyoshi T, Higuchi Y, Itoh T, Kawasaki Y. 2011. Electrophysiological imaging evaluation of schizophrenia and treatment response in Risner MS, ed. Handbook of Schizophrenia Spectrum Disorders,, vol. III Springer.

Sumiyoshi T, Park S, Jayathilake K, Roy A, Ertugrul A, Meltzer HY. 2007a. Effect of buspirone, a serotonin1A partial agonist, on cognitive function in schizophrenia: a randomized, double-blind, placebo-controlled study. Schizophr Res 95: 158-168.

Sumiyoshi T, Suzuki K, Sakamoto H, Yamaguchi N, Mori H, Shiba K, Yokogawa K. 1995. Atypicality of several antipsychotics on the basis of in vivo dopamine- D2 and serotonin-5HT2 receptor occupancy. Neuropsychopharmacology 12: 57-64.

Sumiyoshi T, Matsui M, Yamashita I, Nohara S, Uehara T, Kurachi M, Meltzer HY. 2000. Effect of adjunctive treatment with serotonin-1A agonist tandospirone on memory functions in schizophrenia. J Clin Psychopharmacol 20: 386-388.

Sumiyoshi T, Higuchi Y, Matsui M, Arai H, Takamiya C, Meltzer HY, Kurachi M. 2007b. Effective adjunctive use of tandospirone with perospirone for enhancing verbal memory and quality of life in schizophrenia. Prog Neuropsychopharmacol Biol Psychiatry 31: 965-967.

Sumiyoshi T, Matsui M, Nohara S, Yamashita I, Kurachi M, Sumiyoshi C, Jayathilake K, Meltzer HY. 2001a. Enhancement of cognitive performance in schizophrenia by addition of tandospirone to neuroleptic treatment. Am J Psychiatry 158: 1722-1725.

Sumiyoshi T, Tsunoda M, Higuchi Y, Itoh T, Seo T, Itoh H, Suzuki M, Kurachi M. 2010. Serotonin-1A receptor gene polymorphism and the ability of antipsychotic drugs to improve attention in schizophrenia. Adv Ther 27: 307-313.

Sumiyoshi T, Matsui M, Yamashita I, Nohara S, Kurachi M, Uehara T, Sumiyoshi S, Sumiyoshi C, Meltzer HY. 2001b. The effect of tandospirone, a serotonin(1A) agonist, on memory function in schizophrenia. Biol Psychiatry 49: 861-868.

Sumiyoshi T, Higuchi Y, Itoh T, Matsui M, Arai H, Suzuki M, Kurachi M, Sumiyoshi C, Kawasaki Y. 2009. Effect of perospirone on P300 electrophysiological activity and social cognition in schizophrenia: a three-dimensional analysis with sloreta. Psychiatry Res 172: 180-183.

Uehara T, Sumiyoshi T, Itoh H, Kurata K. 2008. Lactate production and neurotransmitters; evidence from microdialysis studies. Pharmacol Biochem Behav 90: 273-281.

Uehara T, Sumiyoshi T, Matsuoka T, Itoh H, Kurachi M. 2006. Role of 5-HT(1A) receptors in the modulation of stress-induced lactate metabolism in the medial prefrontal cortex and basolateral amygdala. Psychopharmacology (Berl) 186: 218-225.

Uehara T, Sumiyoshi T, Seo T, Itoh H, Matsuoka T, Suzuki M, Kurachi M. 2009. Long-term effects of neonatal MK-801 treatment on prepulse inhibition in young adult rats. Psychopharmacology (Berl) 206: 623-630.

Uehara T, Sumiyoshi T, Seo T, Matsuoka T, Itoh H, Suzuki M, Kurachi M. 2010. Neonatal exposure to MK-801, an N-methyl-D-aspartate receptor antagonist, enhances methamphetamine-induced locomotion and disrupts sensorimotor gating in pre- and postpubertal rats. Brain Res 1352: 223-230.

Uehara T, Itoh H, Matsuoka T, Rujescu D, Genius J, Seo T, Sumiyoshi T. in press. Effect of transient blockade of N-methyl-D-aspartate receptors in the neonatal stage on stress-induced lactate metabolism in medial prefrontal cortex of adult rats; Role of 5-HT1A receptor agonism. Synapse

Wyss MT, Jolivet R, Buck A, Magistretti PJ, Weber B. 2011. In vivo evidence for lactate as a neuronal energy source. J Neurosci 31: 7477-7485.

Yoshino T, Nisijima K, Shioda K, Yui K, Katoh S. 2004. Perospirone, a novel atypical antipsychotic drug, potentiates fluoxetine-induced increases in dopamine levels via multireceptor actions in the rat medial prefrontal cortex. Neurosci Lett 364: 16-21.

8

From Humans to Animals: Animal Models in Schizophrenia

Liesl B. Jones
Lehman College,
CUNY Bronx New York
USA

1. Introduction

Schizophrenia is one of the most devastating psychiatric disorders. Schizophrenia affects 1.1% of the population or 51 million people (NIMH). Schizophrenia is a disorder that affects multiple brain regions and systems. Symptoms include positive symptoms, negative symptoms and cognitive deficits. Much research has focused on two neurotransmitter systems, dopamine and glutamate. Postmortem studies examining morphology have found alterations in dendrites and spines in the prefrontal cortex and the hippocampus, changes in cell number in volume in the thalamus and alterations in protein expression in the prefrontal cortex. Genetic studies have found a number of genes associated with schizophrenia including but not limited to DISC1, neuregulin1, and Dysibindin 1. The current hypothesis based on the postmortem work and genetic studies suggests the etiology of schizophrenia has its origins in development. The changes in dendrites and spines observed in the prefrontal cortex and hippocampus without a change in cell number could occur as a result of alterations in calcium signaling levels in development due to alterations in synaptic input into the prefrontal cortex and hippocampus. The various genes that have been shown to be altered in schizophrenia are also involved in neurodevelopment. DISC1, neuroregulin 1 and Dysbindin 1 have all been shown to be involved in neurite outgrowth and differentiation (Ghiani et al, 2010; Kamiya et al, 2005; Pitcher et al, 2011; Sebat et al., 2009; Wiliams et al., 2010). These data support the above hypothesis that schizophrenia is a neurodevelopmental disorder that may or may not have a genetic predisposition. In order to better understand the etiology of the disease, research needs good models with which to test theory. Genetic models, chemical lesions, and physical lesions have been used to produce animal models to mimic human disorders and are becoming the hallmark of translational research. Animal models in the past have been used to understand how the nervous system develops by using lesions to examine pathways or genetic knockouts to examine the role of genes in development and function of the nervous system. The use of animal models is not limited to basic research but is also used by pharmaceutical companies to test drugs to treat diseases to determine their viability. Whatever their use, animals provide us with a unique way in which to view how the nervous system develops, functions and what happens when development goes wrong. This chapter will focus on the use of animal models as a potential method to study neuropsychiatric disorders.

2. Animal models

Over 50 animal models have been described in the past 30 years (Tseng et al., 2009). The first models tended to be pharmacological constructs linked to dopamine and glutamate. The issue with these models is that they leave out certain aspects of the disorder such as the idea that schizophrenia is a disorder founded in development, cognitive deficits as well as alterations in neuroanatomy and interactions between systems. A review by Harrision (2011) suggests that the problem with modeling schizophrenia is that since it is a disorder that involves so many brain regions, how does one choose a target for the lesion? Schizophrenia therefore, appears to be a disorder involving circuits (Fig 1). One way to choose a target is by picking a brain region shown to be altered anatomically or by choosing a gene whose expression is involved in the development of the structures shown to be altered in schizophrenia. With this in mind two of the most consistent postmortem findings in schizophrenia are lateral ventricular enlargement and a decrease in volume and cell number in the thalamic medial dorsal nucleus. Several models have been designed around these two findings and will be discussed in this chapter. The use of knock out mice to model schizophrenia has also been very popular. The mouse model for Dysbindin 1 has shown much promise in the field of schizophrenia.

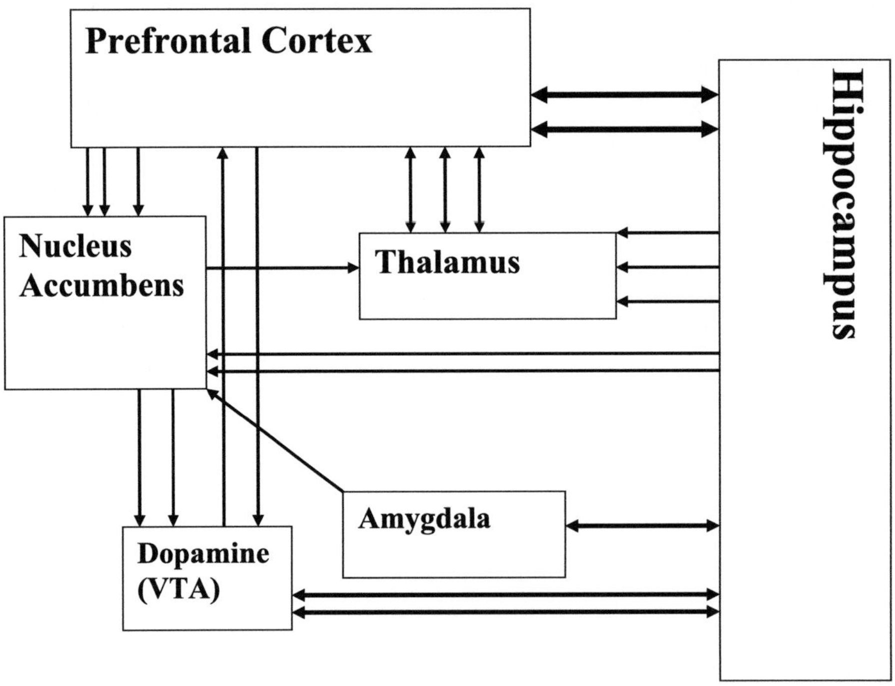

Fig. 1. Schematic showing the circuits thought to be involved in schizophrenia (Tseng et al, 2009).

3. Animal models involving the hippocampus

Lesions of the ventral hippocampus in the rat involve using iobotinic acid to cause a bilateral excitotoxic lesion at postnatal day 7 (Lipska et al, 2002; Becker et al, 1999; Sams-Dodd et al, 1997). One such model involves the neonatal damage of the rat ventral hippocampus; typically, ibotenic acid, causing an excitotoxic lesion, is applied to the ventral hippocampus at postnatal day 7 (Lipska et al 2002; Becker et al, 1999; Sams-Dodd et al, 1997). The animals are allowed to mature and are tested for social interactions (Sams-Dodd et al, 1997), aggression (Becker et al, 1999), and performance in working memory tasks (Lipska et al 2002). This model mimics a spectrum of behavioral features of schizophrenia; it produces functional pathology in other brain regions also implicated in schizophrenia, such as the striatum, the nucleus accumbens, and the prefrontal cortex (PFC). Furthermore, the social and functional effects are not evident until the rat subjects reach adolescence, thus mimicking the timing of onset of symptoms (for review see Lipska, 2004 and Tseng et al, 2009). Following the bilateral lesion at P7 the behaviors emerge in a manner consistent with schizophrenia. Negative symptoms such as aggression and deficits in grooming appear prior to puberty. The cognitive symptoms such as deficits in various types of memory appear at the onset of puberty and the positive symptoms appear late in adolescence (Tseng et al, 2009). This delayed emergence of behaviors mimics that observed in schizophrenia. This model appears to be consistent with many of the behavioral aspects of schizophrenia; however, it lacks construct validity, as schizophrenics do not have a lesion in their hippocampus similar to that seen in the model. Postmortem studies have reported morphometric abnormalities in the hippocampal formation, such as decreased volumes (Falkai & Bogerts, 1986; Heckers et al, 1991) and decreased number of neurons and smaller pyramidal cells in schizophrenia (Falkai & Bogerts, 1986; Jonsson et al, 1999). Other studies have not been able to replicate such findings (Heckers et al, 1991; Walker et al, 2002). Further discrepancy is seen in the morphological evaluation of this model which reports an increase in synaptic density, number of branches, and dendritic length in the pyramidal cells of the PFC (Robinson and Kolb, 1997), which contradicts the compromised morphological evidence in schizophrenia (Byne W et al; 2001, Jones L, Mall N, Byne W; 1998, Bunney WE and Bunney BG; 2000, Schindler MK et al; 2002, Jonsson SAT et al; 1999; Broadbelt et al, 2002, Kalus, 2000; Black et al, 2004; Pierri et al, 2001; Garey et al, 1998; Glantz and Lewis, 2000). Although the discrepancy in anatomical findings between this model and schizophrenia are great, it prevails to be an attractive model because of its implications in the dopaminergic system, a neurotransmitter system known to be affected in this disorder and a major target for therapeutic agents. Recent investigations using this model examined cell excitability in PFC neurons, and it was concluded that the PFC dopamine-glutamate interactions were altered after puberty in the lesioned rats (Tseng et al, 2007). Specifically, the PFC neurons showed enhanced excitability in lesioned animals, which contradicts the common concept of hypofrontality, characteristic of schizophrenic subjects. While the model may have its inconsistencies, the approach using neurodevelopmental damage has merits in developing models for schizophrenia.

The use of excitatory lesions of the entorhinal cortex (EC) has furthered investigation of the effects on the dopaminergic system. It was observed that an EC lesion resulted in the enhancement of methamphetamine-induced dopamine release in the nucleus accumbens and basolateral amygdala (Uehara, et al 2007), implying dysregulation in the dopaminergic neurotransmission in the limbic regions. Although these models offer great insight into circuitry of the dopaminergic system and potential for development of therapeutic agents, it is evident that models based on manipulations of the dopamine system have limited promise. They can imitate a spectrum of schizophrenic behaviors, but they fall short on morphological and physiological findings.

Keeping with the idea that schizophrenia is a disease that affects circuits, another mesiotemporal limbic area used for lesion studies is the amygadala. The amygdala receives projections from the hippocampus and projects to the nucleus accumbens (Fig. 1). A model put forward by Francine Benes examines the effects of altering the circuitry between the amygdala and the hippocampus. The non-competitive GABA-A receptor antagonist picrotoxin was infused into the basolateral complex of the amygdala. This was done to mimic a GABA defect in this region. This model shows alterations in GABAergic neurons in the CA2/3 region of the hippocampus similar to that seen in schizophrenia (Berretta and Benes 2006; Berretta et al, 2009). Daenen et al, (2001) examined several behaviors in rats following a lesion of the amygdala at P7 or P21. The lesions at P7 but not P21 showed alterations in locomotor stereotypy (Daenen et al, 2001) as well as play (Daenen et al, 2002) and exploratory activities (Woletrink et al, 2001). These lesion studies tend to find deficits in social behavior (Becker et al, 1999; Sams-Dodd et al, 1997), working memory (Lipska et al, 2002), and abnormalities in locomotor stereotypy (Daenen et al 2001, 2003). Daenen et al, (2003) also lesioned the ventral hippocampus at P7 and P21 and examined the response to acoustic startle and found that the lesions had no effect on the response to acoustic startle. A final study examined the effect of a mesiotemporal limbic lesion on the expression NAA, a neuronal viability marker in the PFC, and they found a developmental effect in the early-lesioned animals, which was absent from the animals lesioned as adults (Bertolino et al, 1997). In humans, these temporal association areas have widespread connections with the medial dorsal nucleus of the thalamus and the pulvinar nucleus of the thalamus (Byne et al, 2001), which has also been implicated in schizophrenia (Byne et al, 2002; 2001) (Fig. 2). When one looks at the brain regions involved in schizophrenia and the circuits involved, one target region emerges as a location to target in modeling schizophrenia, the medial dorsal nucleus of the thalamus. This nucleus receives multiple inputs from the hippocampus as well as the amygdala and projects to the prefrontal cortex as well as other regions involved in schizophrenia.

4. Animal models and the thalamus

Thalamic association nuclei, such as the medial dorsal nucleus (MD) (Paxinos G, 1986), which have connections to many regions involved in schizophrenia (Paxinos G, 1986; Kuroda et al, 1998), represents an important relevant target for lesion studies (see figure 2).

Normal development of the cerebral cortex is dependent upon reciprocal connections with the thalamus. The close association between the MD and the PFC and EC initiates early in development. The cortical plate differentiates from a densely packed zone of immature cells into lamina, resembling future cortical layers (van Eden 1986); axons from early postmitotic

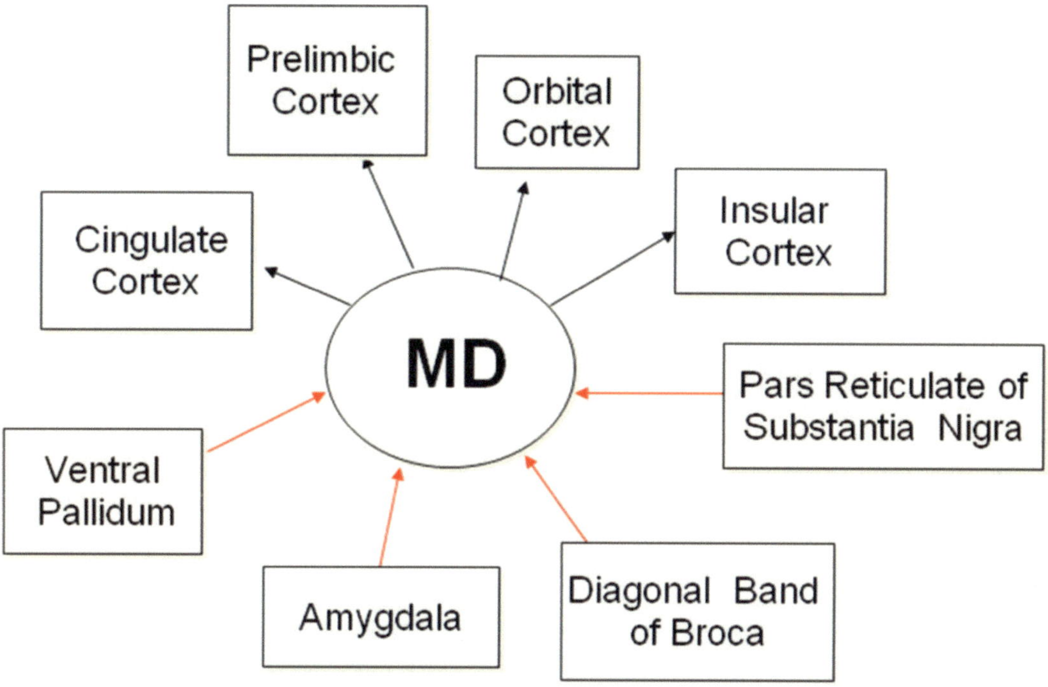

Fig. 2. Circuitry formed by the MD in rats. MD projects to cortex and receives feedback, as well as projections from subcortical structures.

neurons of the cortical subplate pioneer the pathway from the cortex toward subcortical targets, prior to neurons from cortical layers V and VI migrating into position (Molnar 2000). By postnatal day 4 and 5, layer V can be distinguished from the upper cortical plate containing the elements to become layers II and III. The first evidence of retrograde labeling from PFC to MD becomes apparent at this time (Van Eden 1986). The arrival of the MD afferent fibers in the upper cortical plate precedes the completion of layer III differentiation, occurring on postnatal days 9 to 10 (Van Eden 1986). The predominant thalamic input to the PFC is from the medial dorsal nucleus (Negyess et al., 1998, Kuroda 1995a, 1995b). Afferents from the MD synapse on spines and dendritic shafts of pyramidal cells in the PFC (Negyess et al., 1998). Myelination of the axons from the MD to the PFC occurs approximately in the second decade of life (Molnar 2000). Developmental maturation of neurons is activity-dependent (Van Pelt et al., 1996, Kossel et al., 1997, Baker et al., 1997); an early lesion of the MD could therefore result in abnormal development of the PFC. In particular, a decrease in thalamic input to PFC may result in decrease of calcium-mediated stimulation of dendritic remodeling. Binding of glutamate to the N-methyl-D-Aspartate (NMDA) receptor causes an influx of calcium, which triggers the release of calmodulin from the calcium binding protein neurogranin (Ramakers et al., 2001), allowing for calmodulin to bind to calcium. Calcium-calmodulin can activate calcium calmodulin kinase (CaMK) II (Petit et al., 1998), CaM kinase, and CaM Kinases I and IV (Petit et al., 1998). CaMK II has been shown to be important in controlling spine formation (Petit et al., 1998), as well as neuronal arborization, both pre- and post-synaptically (Ramakers et al., 2001, Petit et al., 1998, Kater et al., 1988). CaMK II also phosphorylates MAP2, which in turn promotes dendritic branching.

Dephosphorylation of MAP2 by calcineurin promotes dendritic elongation (Ramakers et al., 2001, Petit et al., 1998, Kater et al., 1988). Current postmortem studies of the PFC have shown a decrease in neurogranin and calmodulin in areas 9 and 32 (Broadbelt et al., 2006, 2008). These data suggest possible alterations in calcium signaling in the PFC. Thus, changes in proteins involved in calcium signaling may lead to changes in dendritic arbors and spines, which are critical to neuronal function, leading to possible alterations in integration of synaptic inputs. Thus information transfer between cells can be altered. In addition, these data suggest that the medial dorsal nucleus is a potential target for a lesion during development that may result in alterations similar to those seen in schizophrenia.

Research has shown that two of the most consistent findings in schizophrenia are volume and cell loss in the MD of the thalamus and enlarged anterior and posterior horns of the lateral ventricles (Pakkenberg; 1990, 1992, Popken et al 2000, Young et al 2000, Byne et al 2001, 2002, Lewis et al 2001). Previous MD lesion studies have primarily looked at the effect of the lesions on behavior (Volk & Lewis 2003; Van Eden et al, 1994; Isseroff et al, 1982). Studies have shown that a lesion of the MD leads to impairments in spatial memory tasks in rats (Isseroff et al, 1982) as well as in monkeys (Aggleton et al., 1983). This spatial memory loss is qualitatively similar to that seen after damage of the prefrontal cortex (Isseroff et al, 1982). MD lesions can also affect working memory as assessed by radial maze tests (Aggleton, 1983; Stokes1990). These findings are consistent with reports of working and spatial memory deficits in schizophrenic patients (Perry et al, 2001). An embryonic animal lesion model for schizophrenia includes intrauterine radiation of rhesus monkeys during thalamic neurogenesis, which results in a 25% loss of thalamic volume, neuron loss, and nonuniform damage to the thalamic complex (Schindler et al, 2002). Although this model is simulating the consistent finding of neuron loss and decreased volume in the thalamus (Pakkenberg; 1990, 1992, Popken et al 2000, Young et al 2000, Byne et al 2001, 2002, Lewis et al 2001), it offers too many variables as the entire fetus is subjected to radiation and thus a spectrum of possible side effects. Several studies showed alterations in working and short-term memory in adult rats following early N-methyl-D-aspartate (NMDA) receptor inhibition in the MD (Garter et al., 1992, Sicar et al., 1998, 2003, Stefani et al., 2005, Wang et al., 2001 for review see Pehrson et al., 2007).

Focusing on the relevant circuitry between the MD and the PFC, one study examined the structural and functional effects of a MD lesion on the PFC in the rat (Van Eden et al, 1998). A study using an electrothermal lesion on the MD on the day of birth analyzed prefrontal architecture on day 35, as well as performance on a delayed alternation task. They found no significant gross changes in the PFC, except for local decreases in cortical width. The behavioral ability in spatial task was also examining the morphology in the PFC; they only examined gross morphology and not specific cellular morphology, which is known to be affected in schizophrenic brains (Garey et al, 1998; Broadbelt et al, 2002; Glantz & Lewis 2000). When using animals as models it is important to understand timing of developmental events. In rats, thalamic fibers grow into the cortex between postnatal day 0 and 7 (Wise et al, 1979), and a lesion performed too early may reflect the plastic ability of the brain. An additional MD lesion study looked at whether an acute excitotoxic lesion of the MD on periadolescent monkeys could produce decreased PFC glutamate decarboxylase mRNA expression (Volk & Lewis, 2003). They found that a substantial lesion did not reduce levels of this GABA-synthesizing enzyme in the PFC four weeks after lesions were performed

(Volk & Lewis, 2003). Their inability to see a change in PFC enzymatic levels may have occurred as a result of the acute lesion in prepubescent animals. The connections between the MD and the PFC may have been well established by the time the lesions were performed, therefore, may not accurately reflect the development. Our laboratory is currently developing an animal model for prefrontal cortical development. Our model is based on the interplay between the prefrontal cortex and the MD and that pyramidal cell development is activity dependent. Our data suggest that the model may also model some of the morphological alterations seen in the prefrontal cortex, such as loss of dendrites and spines, and in the hippocampus, such as change in cell density in CA1. Further work examining behavior needs to be performed to more accurately characterize the model as having relevance for studying schizophrenia.

5. Conclusion

While many of the models discussed reflect the ability to express multiple symptoms of schizophrenia from behavior to genetics to morphology, none of the models appear to mimic all of the symptoms. A current review article by Harrison et al., (2011) suggests that the complexity of the disorder makes it very difficult to accurately model schizophrenia. The authors question how you choose your target for alteration when so many targets appear possible. The point is a valid one, as schizophrenia does not present itself the same way in all individuals. Schizophrenia has many symptoms that can be grouped into three categories: positive, negative and cognitive. Schizophrenics may have symptoms from 1, 2 or all 3 categories. Therefore, it may be very difficult to have one model for all of the symptoms exhibited in schizophrenia. Instead several models may need to be used to understand how schizophrenia manifests itself. What does seem to be consistent in all of the research is the agreement that schizophrenia manifests itself during development, which leads to behavioral alterations in late adolescence and early adulthood that may or may not progress throughout the rest of the individual's life. While one model may not fit all of the symptoms of schizophrenia, it may model enough aspects to help us understand how the disease manifests itself and eventually help us come up with better treatments for a complex disorder which affects over 50 million people.

6. References

Aggleton JP, Mishkin M: Visual recognition impairment following medial thalamic lesions in monkeys. Neuropsychologia. 1983; 21: 189-197.

Baker RE, van Pelt J: Cocultured, but not isolated, cortical explants display normal dendritic development: a long-term quantitative study. Dev Brain Research 1997; 98: 21-29.

Becker A, Grecksch G, Bernstein HG, Hollt V, Bogerts: Social behavior in rats lesioned with ibotenic acid in the hippocampus: quantitative and qualitative analysis. Psychoparmacology 1999; 144: 333-338.

Berretta S, Benes FM: A rat model for neural circuitry abnormalities in schizophrenia. Nature Protocols. 2006; 1: 833-839.

Berretta S, Gisabella B, Benes FM: A rodent model of schizophrenia derived from postmortem studies. Behav. Brain Res. 2009; 204: 363-368.

Black JE, Kodish IM, Grossman AW, Klintsova AY, Orlovskaya D, Vostrikov V, Uranova N, Greenough WT: Pathology of layer V pyramidal neurons in the prefrontal cortex of patients with schizophrenia. Am. J. Psychiatry 2004; 161:742-744.

Broadbelt K, Byne WB, Jones LB: Evidence for a decrease in primary and secondary basilar dendrites on pyramidal cells in area 32 of schizophrenic prefrontal cortex. Schizophrenia Res 2002; 58:75-81.

Broadbelt K, Ramprasaud A, Jones LB: Evidence of altered neurogranin immunoreactivity in areas 9 and 32 of schizophrenic prefrontal cortex. Schizophrenia Res 2006; 87: 6-14.

Broadbelt K, Jones LB: Evidence of altered calmodulin immunoreactivity in areas 9 and 32 of prefrontal schizophrenic prefrontal cortex. J. Psychiatric Research 2008; 42:612-21.

Bubenikova-Valesova V, Horacek J, Vrajova M, Hoschl C: Models of schizophrenia in humans and animals based on inhibition of NMDA receptors. Neurosci. Behav. Reviews 2008; 32:1014-1023.

Bunney We, Bunney BG: Evidence for a compromised dorsolateral prefrontal cortical parallel circuit in schizophrenia. Brain Res. Brain Res. Rev 2000; 31:138-146.

Byne W, Buchsbaum MS, Kemether E, Purohit P, Haroutunian V, Jones L: Postmortem assessment of thalamic nuclear volumes in schizophrenia. Amer J Psychiatry 2001a; 159: 59-65.

Byne W, Buchsbaum MS, Kemether E, Hazlett EA, Shinwari A, Mitropoulou V, Siever LJ: Magnetic resonance imaging of the thalamic mediodorsal nucleus and pulvinar in schizophrenia and schizotypal personality disorder. Arch Gen Psychiatry 2001b; 58:133-140.

Daenen EW, Van der Heyden JA, Kruse CG, Wolterink G, Van Ree JM: Adaptation and habituation to an open field responses to various stressful events in animals with neonatal lesions in the amygdala or ventral hippocampus. Brain Res 2001; 918:153-165.

Daenen EW, Wolterink G, Gerrits MA, Van Ree JM: The effects of neonatal lesions in the amygdala or ventral hippocampus on social behaviour later in life. Behav. Brain Res. 2002; 136: 571-582.

Daenen EW, Wolterink G, Van Der Heyden JA, Kruse CG, Van Ree JM: Neonatal lesions in the amygdala or ventral hippocampus disrupt prepulse inhibition of the acoustic startle response; implications for an animal model of neurodevelopmental disorders like schizophrenia. Eur Neuropsychopharmacol. 2003; 13:187-97.

Falkai P, Bogerts B: Cell loss in the hippocampus of schizophrenics. Eur. Arch. Psychiatry Neurol. Sci. 1986; 236: 154-161.

Garey LJ., Ong WY., Patel TS., Kanani M., Davis A., Mortimer AM., Barnes TR., Hirsch SR: Reduced dendritic spine density on cerebral cortical pyramidal neurons in schizophrenia. Journal Neurology Neurosurgery Psychiatry 1998; 65:446-453.

Garter JA, de Bruin JP: Chronic neonatal MK- 801 treatment results in an impairment of spatial learning in the adult rat. Brain Res 1992; 580: 12-17.

Glantz LA., Lewis DA: Decreased dendritic spine density on prefrontal cortical pyramidal neurons in schizophrenia. Arch. Gen. Psych. 2000; 57:65-73.

Ghiani CA, Starcevic M, Rodriguez-Fernandez IA, Nazarian R, Cheli VT, Chan LN, Malvar JS, de Vellis J, Sabatti C, Dell'Angelica EC: The dysbindin-containing complex (BLOC-1) in brain: developmental regulation, interaction with SNARE proteins, and role in neurite outgrowth. Mol. Psych. 2010; 15: 204-215.

Harrison Lm, Mair RG: A comparison of the effects of frontal cortical and thalamic lesions on measures of spatial learning and memory in the rat. Behav Brain Research 1996; 75: 195-206.

Harrison PJ., Pritchett D., Stumpenhorst K., Betts JF., Nissen W, Schweimer J., Lane T., Philip W.J. Burnet PWJ., Lamsa KP., Sharp T., Bannerman DM., Tunbridge EM: Genetic mouse models relevant to schizophrenia: Taking stock and looking forward. (2011). Neuropharmacology; 1-4.

Heckers S, Heisen H, Geiger B, Beckmann H: Hippocampul neuron number in schizophrenia. A stereological study. Arch. Gen. Psychiatry 1991; 48: 1002-1008.

Isseroff A, Rosvold HE, Galkin TW, Goldman-Rakic PS: Spatial memory impairments following damage to the mediodorsal nucleus of the thalamus in rhesus monkeys. Brain Research 1982; 232: 97-113.

Jones L, Johnson N, Byne W: Alterations in MAP2 staining in area 9 and 32 of schizophrenic prefrontal cortex. Psychiatry Res. 2002; 114: 137-148.

Jonsson SA, Luts A, Guldberg-Kjaer N, Ohman R: Pyramidal neuron size in the hippocampus of schizophrenics correlates with total cell count and degree of cell disarray. Eur. Arch. Psychiatry Clin. Neurosci. 1999; 249:169-173.

Kalus P, Muller TJ, Zuschratter W, Senitz D: The denrtitic architecture of prefrontal pyramidal neurons in schizophrenic patients. Neuroreport 2000; 11:3621-3625.

Kamiya A, Kubo K-i, Tomoda T, Takaki M, Youn R, Ozeki Y, Sawamura N, Park U, Kudo C, Okawa M, Ross CA, Hatten ME, Nakajima K, Sawa A: A schizophrenia-associated mutation of DISC1 perturbs cerebral cortex development. Nature Cell Bio. 2005; 7: 1167-1178.

Kater SB, Mattson MP, Cohan C, Connor J: Calcium regulation of the neuronal growth cone. Trends Neuroscience 1988; 11:315-321.

Kossel AH, Williams CV, Schweizer M, Kater SB: Afferent innervation influences the development of dendritic branch and spines via both activity-dependent and non-activity-dependent mechanisms. J Neuroscience 1997; 17: 6314-6324.

Kuroda M, Murakami K, Kishi K, Price JL: Thalamic synapses between axons from the mediodorsal thalamic nucleus and pyramidal cells in the prelimbic cortex of the rat. J Comp Neurology 1995; 356:143-151.

Kuroda M, Murakami K, Shinkai M, Ojima H, Kishi K: Electron microscopic evidence that axon terminals from the mediodorsal thalamic nucleus make direct synaptic contacts with callosal cells in the prelimbic cortex of the rat. Brain Research 1995; 677: 348-353.

Kuroda M, Yokofujita J, Murakami K: An ultrastructural study of the neural circuit between the prefrontal cortex and the mediodorsal nucleus of the thalamus. Progress Neurobiology 1998; 54: 417-458.

Lipska BK: Using animal models to tes a neurodevelopmentla hypothesis of schizophrenia. J. Psychiatry Neurosci. 2004; 29: 282-286.

Lipska BK, Weinberger DR: A neurodevelopmental model of schizophrenia: neonatal disconnection of the hippocampus. (2002). Neurotox Res; 4: 469-475.

Molnar Z: Development and evolution of thalamocortical interactions. Eur J Morphology 2000; 38(5): 313-320.

Negyessy L, Hámori J, Bentivoglio M: Contralateral cortical projection to the mediodorsal thalamic nucleus: origin and synaptic organization in the rat. Neuroscience 1998; 84(3):741-53.

Pakkenberg B: Pronounced *reduction* of total neuron number in mediodorsal thalamic nucleus and nucleus accumbens in schizophrenics. *Arch Gen Psychiatry* 1990; 47:1023-1028.

Pakkenberg B: The volume of the medial dorsal thalamic nucleus in treated and untreated schizophrenics. Schizophrenia Research 1992; 7:95-100.

Paxinos G, Kus L, Ashwell KWS, Watson C: Chemoarchitectonic atlas of the rat forebrain. London. Academic Press 1999.

Paxinos G, Watson C: The rat brain in stereotaxic Coordinates. Sydney Academic Press 1986.

Pehrson A.l, Walenting DM, Wood JT, Vinck SA, Porter JH: Early postnatal antagonism of glutametergic NMDA receptors impairs reference and working memory performances, but has no effect on locomotor activity in male C57Bl/6 mice. 2007; 18:S1-S11.

Perry W, Minassian A, Feifel D, Braff DL: Sensorimotor gating deficits in bipolar disorder patients with acute psychotic mania. Biol. Psychiatry 2001; 50:418-424.

Petit TL, LeBoutillier JC, Gregorio A, Libstug H: The pattern of dendritic development in the cerebral cortex of the rat. Dev Brain Research 1988; 41:209-219.

Pierri JN, Volk CL, Auh S, Sampson A, Lewis DA: Decreased somal size of deep layer 3 pyramidal neurons in the prefrontal cortex of subjects with schizophrenia. Arch Gen. Psychiatry 2001; 58:466-473.

Pitcher GM, Kalia LV, Ng D, Goodfellow NM, Yee KT, Lambe EK, Salter MW: Schizophrenia susceptibility pathway neuregulin 1–ErbB4 suppresses Src upregulation of NMDA receptors. Nature Medicine. 2011; 17:470-478.

Popken GJ, Bunney WE Jr, Potkin SG, Jones EG: Subnucleus-specific loss of neurons in medial thalamus of schizophrenics. Proc Natl Acad Science USA 2000; 97: 9276-9280.

Ramakers GJA, Avci B, van Hulten P, van Ooyen A, van Pelt J, Pool CW, Lequin MB: The role of calcium signaling in early axonal and dendritic morphogenesis of rat cerebral cortex neurons under non-stimulated growth conditions. Dev Brain Research 2001; 126: 163-172.

Robinson TE, Kolb: Persistent structural modifications in nucleus accumbens and prefrontal cortex neurons produced by previous experience with amphetamine. J. Neuroscie 1997; 17:8491-8497.

Sams-Dodd F, Lipska BK, Weinberger DR: Neonatal lesions of the rat ventral hippocampus result in hyperlocomotion and deficits in social behavior in adulthood. 1997; Psychopharmacology 132; 303-310.

Schindler MK, Wang L, Selemon LD, Goldman-Rakic PS, Rakic P, Csernansky JG: Abnormalities of thalamic volume and shape detected in fetally irradiated rhesus monkeys with high dimensional brain mapping. Biol. Psychiatry 2002; 51:827-837.

Sebat J, Levy DL, McCarthy SE. Rare structural variants in schizophrenia: one disorder, multiple mutations; one mutation, multiple disorders. Trends Genet 2009; 25: 528–35.

Sinopoli KJ, Floresco SB, Galea LAM: Systemic and local administration of estrdiol into the prefrontal cortex or hippocampus differentially alters working memory. Neruobio. Learning Memory 2006; 86:293-304.

Sircar R: Postnatal phencyclidine-induced deficits in adult water maze performance is associated with N-methyl-D-aspartate receptoer upregulation. Int. J. Dev. Neurosci. 2003; 21:159-167.

Sircar R, Rudy JW: Repeated neonatal phencyclidine treatment impairs performance of a spatial table in juvenile rats. Ann. NY. Acad. Sci 1998; 844: 303-309.

Stefani MR, Moghaddam B: Transient N-methyl-D-sparttr recepter blockade in early develoment causes lasting cognitive deficits relevant to schizophrenia. Biol. Psychiatry 2005; 57:433-436.

Stokes KA, Best PJ: Mediodorsal thalamic lesions impair "reference" and "working" memory in rats. Physiol Behavior 1990; 47: 471-476.

Tseng K, Chambers RA, Lipska B: Neonatal ventral hippocampul lesion as a heuristic neurodevelopmentalmodel of schizophrenia. Brain Beh. Res. 2009; 204: 295-305.

Tseng KY, Lewis BL, Lipska BK, O'Donnell P: Post-pubertal disruption of medial prefrontal cortical dopamine-glutamate interactions in a developmental animal model of schizophrenia. Bio. Psychiatry 2007; 62: 730-738.

Uehara T, Sumiyoshi T, Matsuoka T, Itoh H, Kurachi M: Effect of prefrontal cortex inactivation on behavioral and neurochemical abnormalities in rats with excitotoxic lesions of the entorhinal cortex. Synapse 2007; 61:391-400.

Van Eden CG: Development of connections between the mediodorsal nucleus of the thalamus and the prefrontal cortex in the rat. J Comp Neurol. 1986; 244:349-59.

Van Pelt J, van Ooyen A, Corner MA: Growth cone dynamics and activity-dependent processes in neuronal network development. Progress Brain Research 1996; 108: 333-346.

Volk DW, Lewis DA: Effects of a mediodorsal thalamus lesion on prefrontal inhibitory circuitry: implications for schizophrenia. Biol. Psychiatry. 2003; 53:385-389.

Wang C, McInnis J, Ross-Sanchez M, Shinnick-Gallagheere P, Wiley JL, Johnson K M: Long-term behavioral and neurodegenerative effects of perinatal phencyclidine adminstration: implications for schizophrenia. Neurosci. 2001; 107:535-550.

Williams NM, Zaharieva I, Martin A, Langley K, Mantripragada K, Fossdal R,et al. Rare chromosomal deletions and duplications are associated with attention deficit hyperactivity disorder and overlap with those conferring susceptibility to autism and schizophrenia. Lancet 2010; 376: 1401–8.

Wise SP, Fleshman JW, Jones EG: Maturation of pyramidal cell form in relation to developing afferent and efferent connections of the rat somatic sensory cortex. J Neuroscience 1979; 4:1275-1297.

Wolterink G, Daenen LE, Dubbeldam S, Gerrits MA, van Rijn R, Kruse CG, Van Der Heijden JA Van Ree JM: Early amygdala damage in the rat as a model for neurodevelopmental psychopathological disorders. Eur. Neuropsycopharmacol 2001; 11:51-59.

Young KA, Manaye KF, Liang C-L, Hicks PB, German DC: Reduced numbers of mediodorsal and anterior thalamic neurons in schizophrenia. Biol Psychiatry 2000; 47: 944-953.

9

Behavioral Tests for Evaluation of Information Processing and Cognitive Deficits in Rodent Animal Models of Neuropsychiatric Disorders

Ales Stuchlik, Tomas Petrasek, Hana Hatalová, Lukas Rambousek, Tereza Nekovarova and Karel Vales
Institute of Physiology, Academy of Sciences
Czech Republic

1. Introduction

Neuropsychiatric disorders represent a serious medical and human issue. In general, these diseases are detrimental to the quality of life and sociability of afflicted patients. Moreover, they are an immense socio-economic burden. Brain disorders are sometimes denoted as ´graveyards of pharmaceutical enterprises´, referring to relatively a large proportion of drugs for these diseases failing to prove efficient or safe in later phases of clinical trials. Our understanding of what really happens in the central nervous system (CNS) is very limited, especially in relation to normal and pathological behaviors. This limitation also effects the research of neuropsychiatric disorders. We do not know the exact pathogenic mechanisms of numerous diseases, such as Alzheimer's disease or schizophrenia, which prevents the causal treatment of many of them. The symptomatic-like treatment often yields an insufficient therapeutic outcome and in many cases, is accompanied by serious side-effects (as is the case for classical antipsychotics in refractory schizophrenic patients). In some areas of neuro-science research, we are often just beginning to understand brain-behavior relationships in health and disease.

Aside from being a serious socio-economic and human challenge, many neuropsychiatric disorders involve deficits in mental and behavioral functions. These often reflect disrupted processing of information in the brain (such as gating deficits; more later), storage of information (learning and memory deficits, extending from working memory to long-term retention) and higher cognitive domains (such as impaired executive functions, cognitive control deficits). The diseased brain seems to process at least some information incorrectly, which contributes to the manifestation of the disease and may seriously alter behavior and the normal functioning of afflicted patients. Therefore, beside basic studies aimed at the nature of information processing and cognition impairments in human CNS diseases, important usage of behavioral tests lies in both screening for putative cognition-improving drugs and cognitive side-effects of established and novel pharmaceuticals.

Behavioral researchers in pre-clinical research conventionally use tests of information processing and sensorimotor gating, often tested with prepulse inhibition of the startle reflex (e.g. Bubenikova-Valesova et al., 2007), spontaneous behaviors (e.g. Palenicek et al.,

2007), latent inhibition tests and many others. In addition, not only memory scientists but also application-oriented researchers have often sought to examine higher mechanisms of cognition, such as spatial navigation and its changes in animal models and even in human patients (e.g. Hort et al., 2007). Moreover, spatial navigation to hidden goals (place navigation) has attracted much attention as a possible animal model of declarative memory (O´Keefe and Nadel, 1978). This is the domain traditionally ascribed only to humans representing the conscious remembering of facts and events.

This chapter will present some established tests in gating and information processing as well as several learning, memory and cognition tests. Beside sections dedicated to classical spatial navigation tests (i.e., the Morris water maze and radial maze), we will present some past and recent behavioral tests of navigation in dynamic environments and cognitive coordination and discuss their usage in animal models.

2. Animal models

Animal models of neuropsychiatric disorders represent an extremely useful approach in the research of both the neurobiology and treatment of CNS disease. When considering CNS diseases, animal models can be defined as (usually experimental) interventions into CNS or brain function. These manipulations often project specific and unusual behaviors. These may be straightforward hyperlocomotion in a pharmacological model of schizophrenia induced by NMDA receptor antagonists or compulsive adherence to specific routes and objects in animal models of obsessive-compulsive disorder (OCD induced by repeated systemic treatment with quinpirole, a D2-like receptor agonist. (Szechtman et al., 2001, Dvorkin et al., 2008; Dvorkin et al., 2010; Woody and Szechtman, 2011). Nevertheless, they should not be anthropomorphized (such as a *´diseased rat´*) but have the purpose to serve as model reproductions in laboratory animals of specific classes of symptoms of CNS disorders, rather than a disorder as a whole, despite common usage of the term of animal models in the latter .

It is obviously impossible to reproduce the full symptomatic and causal spectrum of human neuropsychiatric disorders in laboratory animals. However, results from these models allow for investigating potentially beneficial drugs, beside often significantly contributing to the understanding of the disease. Animal models of neuropsychiatric disorders are usually evaluated according to criteria of validities. The ´resemblance' between the animal model and human pathological phenotypes is usually termed as *face validity*, related to similar pathophysiology and strong phenomenological similarities between (often aberrant) behaviors of an animal and specific symptoms of the human condition. Evaluation of whether the different behavior in different species reflects similar underlying processes is a question of construct validity (Ellenbroek and Cools, 1990). In general, the *construct validity* refers to a correlation between the theorized outcome of measuring and measuring itself. Construct validity is therefore more relevant, as it relates to similarity in the underlying neurobiological mechanisms that are involved in particular behavior. The precise expression of the behavior could be different in human and in experimental animal models. The concept of construct validity is closely related to etiological validity. A model shows etiological validity if the etiology of the disease in the human and animal model is the same (Tordjman et al., 2007). However, to model particular psychopathology it is necessary to specify which is the core process postulated to be common to the disorder and to the model.

It is difficult to assess etiological validity for complex human disorders, such as neuropsychiatric disorders, because so little is known about the etiology of the illness. *Predictive validity* generally refers to the extent to which the outcome of one measurement predicts the outcome of another measurement or some other criterion. In biomedical research, it refers to the predictive value that observations made in animals could have for the conditions in humans. It can be applied to various situations, but in practice, the predictive validity of animal models in psychopharmacology is primarily used in a narrow sense to refer to the ability of a model to identify drugs with potentially therapeutic value for humans. (Wilner, 1991). Reliability applies to the accuracy with which the observations, both clinical and experimental, are made.

Together with other human disorders, neuropsychiatric disorders and especially accompanying deficits in information processing and cognition share the urgent necessity to find appropriate and sensitive animal models even if limited. Nevertheless, because the neuropsychiatric disorders affect mostly features and conditions considered as typically human, the modeling of psychiatric conditions could be the most difficult and cannot be reproduced exactly in the rodents. However, there is hope for more specific behavioral approaches which can be used in any rodent animal models of cognitive disruption and which will be presented in the main chapter.

2.1 Tests of sensorimotor gating

Deficits in gating functions and signal processing are often found in neuropsychiatric disorders and their animal models. It has been proposed that they might contribute to impaired cognitive functions. The topic has been covered by a number of excellent reviews (e.g. Geyer 2008, Swerdlow et al., 2008; Castagné et al., 2009). A classic example of the gating paradigm is auditory *´sensory gating´*, in which two audible pulses (clicks) are presented to a subject in a conditioning-testing manner and its P50 event-related potentials are measured (Adler et al., 1982; Adler et al., 1986; Martin et al., 2004; Martin and Freedman, 2007). In normal subjects (both rats and humans), the potential response to the second stimulus is diminished (Adler et al., 1982; Adler et al., 1986), reflecting insufficient habituation (reviewed in Geyer, 2008). It was demonstrated that a deficit in this sensory gating was present in schizophrenia patients (Adler et al., 1982) and in rats in the animal model of schizophrenia (Adler et al., 1986). Moreover, this phenomenon is also disrupted in manic patients with bipolar disorder (Franks et al., 1986; Baker et al., 1990). This paradigm also significantly contributed to the concept of the beneficial effects of alpha-7 nicotinic agonists in schizophrenia (Martin et al., 2004; Martin and Freedman, 2007).

Perhaps the widest testing of sensorimotor gating as a measure of information processing is the prepulse inhibition (PPI) of the startle reflex, elicited by a strong sensory stimulus, usually a sound, but other sensory modalities may be considered as well. Since the test involves a motor component (startle reflex), it can be viewed as a true *sensorimotor* gating paradigm. If the prepulse (which is not capable of eliciting a startle reaction) is presented at an appropriate interval (usually 30-500ms) before the pulse, subsequent reduction of the startle due to a prepulse is considered a measure of sensorimotor gating. Its disruption (meaning that subject exhibit strong startle reaction even after administration of both prepulse and pulse) is found in several CNS disorders such as Alzheimer's disease (Hejl et al., 2004; Ueki et al., 2006), schizophrenia (Braff et al., 1992; van den Buuse, 2010; reviewed in

Braff and Geyer, 1990), and bipolar disorder (Rich et al., 2005; Giakoumaki et al., 2006), but reports have been published also on disrupted PPI in obsessive-compulsive disorder (OCD; Hoenig et al., 2005) or attention deficit/hyperactivity disorder (ADHD; Castellanos et al., 1996; Conzelmann et al., 2010).

Perhaps the most abundant usage of the PPI test in humans and animals relates to schizophrenia. It was proposed that deficits in information processing and the impaired ability to distinguish between irrelevant and relevant information belongs to core symptoms of this disease (Ellenbroek and Cools, 1990). As the test is fully applicable to both rats and humans, it allows direct comparison of sensorimotor gating deficits in human patients and laboratory animals. In animal models of CNS disorders, an experimental disruption of PPI is usually induced by pharmacological or neurodevelopmental manipulations. The PPI is disrupted after application of dopamine agonists, such as apomorphine and amphetamine (Mansbach et al., 1998; Auclair et al., 2006), N-methyl-D-aspartate (NMDA) receptor antagonists such as ketamine, phencyclidine or MK-801 (Mansbach and Geyer, 1989; de Bruin et al., 1999; Bubenikova et al., 2005a; Bubenikova-Valesova et al., 2007), but interestingly also after treatment with MDMA (Bubenikova et al., 2005b), serotonergic hallucinogens (Ouagazzal et al., 2001; Palenicek et al., 2008) or scopolamine (Jones and Shannon, 2000; Thomsen et al., 2010). Neurodevelopmental procedures such as isolated rearing (Geyer et al., 1993; Bakshi et al., 1998), maternal deprivation (Ellenbroek et al., 1998; Ellenbroek and Cools, 2000) and neonatal lesions of the ventral hippocampus (Sams-Dodd et al., 1997; Len Pen and Moreau, 2002) also affect this phenomenon. These changes in animal models can be, in some cases, reversed by anti-psychotic treatment (e.g. Bakshi et al., 1998; Len Pen and Moreau, 2002; Bubenikova et al., 2005a). PPI can be also successfully applied to genetically modified mice in animal models (Geyer et al., 2002; Powell et al., 2009).

When considering the usefulness of PPI in animal models of schizophrenia and other psychiatric disorders, one must consider several important points. The PPI paradigm is fully translational, i.e., it can be feasibly used both in laboratory rodents and humans, which facilitates direct comparison of gating deficits in human CNS disorders and their animal models. This is a significant advantage of the test, although it is not the only translatable task out of the plethora of tests used in animal models. The test is also quite simple and basic gating deficits can be expected to reflect complex impairments of informational processing, which may lead to cognitive deficit. However, when interpreting the results of PPI experiments, it should be emphasized that the test is perhaps too simple to reveal memory or cognitive impairments. In memory terms, PPI is essentially a modification of reflex behavior (startle). Despite this limitation, the prepulse inhibition of the startle reflex is abundantly used and a very informative behavioral paradigm for gating mechanisms studied in animal models of CNS disorders.

2.2 Behavioral tests of learning, memory and cognitive functions

Behavioral tests for the assessment of learning and memory (and other types of cognitive domains, such a the cognitive coordination, more later) belong to powerful tools in the hands of researchers focused on animal models of neuropsychiatric disorders, their brain and behavioral deficits. They have also significance for scientists focused on procognitive drugs. Beside these functions, spatial orientation or place navigation (i.e., navigation to directly imperceptible goals) belong to central models for studying cognitive deficits in experimental animals. Navigation to (or away from) invisible goals can be provided by two complementary processes: allothetic (allocentric) and idiothetic (egocentric) orientation (Mittelstaedt and Mittelstaedt., 1980; Mittelstaedt and Glasauer, 1991). Many forms of spatial navigation depend on the hippocampus both in rats (Morris et al., 1982) and humans (Maguire et al., 2006). Indeed, neurons exist in the hippocampus and interconnected structures of rodents that produce firing depending on complex environmental features such as spatial position (place cells, O'Keefe and Dostrovsky, 1971), or direction (head direction cells, Taube et al., 1990a,b). Other important cell types such as grid cells in the medial entorhinal cortex (Hafting et al., 2005), border cells (Solstad et al., 2008), boundary vector cells (Level et al., 2009), goal cells (Hok et al., 2005; 2007) and others, as well as neurons with mixed properties, have recently been discovered.

The following sections will present several selected tests of learning and memory which were tested or have promising potential in the research of pre-clinical animal models. Our selection must be subjective. Many important tests are reviewed elsewhere in scientific literature. Every test is presented in the context of the specific behavioral function that it involves and the significance for the study of animal models is at least briefly discussed.

2.2.1 Morris Water Maze (MWM)

The Morris water maze (MWM) is the classic, and probably most widely used test of spatial learning and memory. The apparatus was designed by Richard G. Morris in 1981 (Morris, 1981, Morris, 1984). It represents a circular maze with larger diameter (e.g. 180 cm), filled with opaque water, in which a rodent (typically a rat), released from various locations on the pool periphery, searches for an escape platform hidden under the water surface. The trial usually stops either when a rat has found the platform, or after a defined maximum duration is completed (e.g. 60 s), after which the animal is gently guided to it. In any case the animal is allowed to stay on the platform for fixed period of time (e.g. 15 s). This test is unique in that virtually all proximal (olfactory etc.) cues are hidden (the animal swims in the water) and only the distal, landmarks outside a pool can be used to localize the platform in a ´cognitive map-like´ fashion (in the classical version). In addition, the test uses the natural ability of rats to swim while not causing a major distress to the animals despite a significant stress response induced by the task (Hölscher, 1999; D´Hooge and De Deyn, 2001). Another advantage of the test is its simplicity; which has contributed significantly to its success and massive use. The behavior of rats in the Morris water maze can be evaluated by many criteria. Beside *escape latency*, i.e., the time needed to find the platform, swim speed and path length should be analyzed in order to control for this factor, which may also provide an indication of sensorimotor or motivational impairments. In many cases, the total path to the platform provides a better solution than escape latency. It is also preferred to use a measure of thigmotaxis, such as time spent at the wall. This has proven to be very useful in assessing behavioral strategies in these tests (e.g. Garthe et al., 2009). There are a number of other measures, including direction angle, Whishaw error etc., which are reviewed elsewhere. Generally the design, use and aspects of the MWM has been reviewed in several papers (e.g. McNamara and Skelton, 1993; D´Hooge and De Deyn, 2001; Clark and Martin, 2005).

The Morris water maze is typically used in two basic experimental protocols: *The reference (or long-term) memory version (also incremental version or place version;* reviewed in Clark and

Martin, 2005) involves the training of rats released from the periphery of the pool to find a hidden platform, the position of which is stable across daily sessions. There are usually more swims (trials) in daily sessions, e.g. 8, 10 or 12. The learning in this task is incremental, and healthy animals of the Long-Evans strain from the breeding colony of the Institute of Physiology, AS CR usually reach the asymptote escape latency by the fourth daily session (with 8 swims; Stuchlik et al., 2004; Vales et al., 2006; Stuchlik et al., 2007a). An early study by Morris showed that place navigation in this version is impaired by a hippocampal lesion. However, this version can also be made hippocampus-independent as well as resistant to several pharmacological manipulations after extensive pre-training or specific training protocols. An interesting procedure is the so-called non-spatial pre-training (NSP; Saucier et al., 1996; Cain et al., 1997) in which animals are first made familiar with all procedural aspects of the task (´rules´), such as that the platform is in the maze. There is no way to get on the wall etc. The pre-training is usually pursued by closing a dark curtain (without any cues) around the pool and putting the submerged platform in random places in the pool. Animals thus get fully acquainted with searching for the platform, but do not know where to search. Such pre-training was found to eliminate a number of deficits, such as after NMDA receptor and cholinergic blockade (Saucier et al., 1996; Cain et al., 1997), serotonin depletion (Beiko et al., 1997) or diazepam treatment (Cain, 1997).

Another variant of the Morris water maze task is a *delayed-matching-to place version* (DMP; Steele and Morris et al., 1999, O'Carroll et al., 2006), in which animals are released in four trials a day and the platform position is changed between days (but always stays the same within four trials in a particular day). Therefore, the rat cannot locate the platform correctly or find it just by chance in the first swim every day. However, a second swim already contains a memory trace from the first one and typically this swim is evaluated. Moreover, multiple inter-trial intervals (ITIs) between the first and second swims can be used (e.g. 15s; 20min and 90 min). There should be no interference between positions in particular days, i.e. each position should be used only once. The task represents a paradigm for the assessment of one-trial spatial learning. With short delays (e.g. 15 s), this modification is essentially a test of spatial working memory and longer delays may be used for evaluating the persistence of the memory trace (O'Carroll et al., 2006). The DMP test in the Morris water maze is strictly hippocampus-dependent, meaning that animals with a hippocampal lesion were not capable of improving from the first to the second swim and thus failed to learn (Steele and Morris, 1999) even after extensive experience with the maze.

The Morris water maze, as in other learning and memory tasks, requires a control for a confounding effect of a more general impairment, such as in perceptual, motivational and procedural functions. This can be tested by a control test, visible platform test, in which the platform is raised above the water and animals are allowed directly to it. Moreover, performance in the spatial versions should be well analyzed for sensorimotor and other measures in order to detect a ´non-cognitive impairment.´ After completion of the whole training or even after each daily session (Markowska et al., 1993), a ´probe trial´ may be performed, during which a rat is allowed to swim freely in the pool and to show a potential preference for a given zone, e.g. time in cardinal quadrants of the maze or number of crossings through the previous platform location. Scientists sometimes use various and more sophisticated designs of the basic MWM configurations, with analyses of behavioral strategies (e.g. Garthe et al., 2009).

The MWM has become a benchmark test for learning and memory deficits in animal models and preclinical research in general. In the context of the use of this test, it might be emphasized that there are also other modifications and protocols including a ´working memory version´ (e.g. eight swims daily with the target position changed between days (Rezacova et al., 2011))- However, this might be confounded by long-term memory, versions using insets (annular water maze), versions with on-demand or an Atlantis platform (Buresova et al., 1985; Spooner et al., 1994) and some studies aiming at an assessment of ´self-motion´ or ´idiothetic´ navigation (Moghaddam and Bures, 1996;1997) or path integration (Benhamou, 1997) in the MWM. Testing of the working memory in the MWM is required due to information processing and working memory deficits in many CNS disorders, such as schizophrenia (e.g. Van Snellenberg, 2009).

A relevant notion for animal models in the MWM is the influential and strongly corroborated concept that the MWM does not undergo systems consolidation, supported by the fact that hippocampus ablations disrupted the memory in the MWM any time after acquisition, both for recent and remote memories (Clark et al., 2005; Martin et al., 2005, Broadbent et al., 2006), which contradicts the view of a transfer of memory trace from hippocampus to neocortical areas, at least in this task (reviewed in Kubik et al., 2007). Athough, the test is widely used to assess the properties of established potential antipsychotics in animal models of schizophrenia (Bubenikova-Valesova et al., 2008a,b; van der Staay et al., 2011; reviewed in Castagné et al., 2009), antipsychotic drugs impair memory in the Morris water maze in naive rats (Skarsfeldt, 1996).

2.2.2 Radial maze

The radial maze (or radial-arm maze) is a classic behavioral test employing spatial cognition as a model for the study of memory, learning and the effects of drugs or gene manipulation. The method is a standard of spatial memory research. The maze was invented by Olton and Samuelson in 1976 (Olton and Samuelson, 1976). This task rapidly became popular and widely used in behavioral neuroscience research. In the original version, the maze had a central octagonal platform and eight arms of the same length. The ´standard version´ of the maze, which is conventionally used, consists of a platform and identical arms radiating from the platform spaced at regular angles - the number of arms is usually eight, but other versions are used as well: e.g. four arms - this maze is known as the ´plus maze´ (Zeldin and Olton, 1986); twelve arms (Cook et al., 1985), seventeen or even twenty four (Buresova and Bures, 1982). The radial maze apparatus is commonly elevated above the floor and placed in a room with many salient visual cues that can be used for allothetic orientation. In the standard version, similar to the initial Olton experiment, the maze is fully baited, which means that at the end of each arm are placed food rewards. An animal has a limited time or an amount of choices, therefore the optimal strategy in a fully baited maze is to visit every arm only once. There are numerous interesting modifications of the radial maze, such as an aquatic version using aversive stimuli rather than appetitive stimuli (Buresova et al., 1985), or a version combining but dissociating both *win-shift* and *win-stay* strategies (Packard et al., 1989).

Many parameters can be used to evaluate behavior and memory in particular in the radial maze - the fundamental and the most apparent is the number of errors. We define an error as a return of the rat to the previously visited arm. Another parameter is the rank of the first error - the number of consecutive correct responses before an error occurs. These two parameters evaluate the efficiency of animals in the test. With training the number of errors decreases and the rank of the first error increases. To illustrate not only their efficacy but also their strategies, it is possible to quantify the angles between two successfully visited arms (Dubreuil et al., 2003). Another parameter is the degree of divergence (Ammassari-Teule and Caprioli, 1985), which is counted only for successful trials with no errors, and the degree of difference is counted as the number of arms between two subsequent correct choices plus one. The number could be averaged for trials during the whole daily session. Degree of divergence equals 7 if rats are using a clockwise strategy, which means they visit systematically all 8 arms. Other parameters include e.g. the sequential position of error which determines relative probability of repetition of choice (Olton and Samuelson, 1976). For each animal and each day, the first seven choices are ordered (the eighth choice is not considered because after this choice the session is ended and there is no opportunity to repeat a choice). The observed relative probability of repeating the correct choice is calculated. Scores could range from 0 to 100 percent. 100 percent indicates that all errors are made by repeating this position, 0 percent indicates that this choice was not repeated. The results show that animals have the tendency to make errors in the arm they chose at the beginning of the session. In the original Olton version all arms were initially open and rats could freely explore all of them without any restrictions.

In the late seventies, Olton and his colleagues introduced a new version of the task with inter-choice time intervals, where the access to the arms is prevented (confinement intervals) (Olton, 1979; Olton et al., 1980). Olton implemented this step to prevent rats from stereotypic behavior which he observed. However, the literature reports the use of both versions of the radial maze: with and without confinement. Dubreuil systematically tested the performance of rats in the maze without and with confinements of different durations (Dubreuil et al., 2003). They found that both groups - without confinement and with confinement of 10sec. reached a similar efficiency after 12 days of training, although the confinement group made more errors during the training. However, even with a similar level performance rats from a different group could use different behavioral strategies to solve the task. The rats from the no-confinement group used (at least in some sessions) a clockwise strategy, thus they visited, systematically, all the arms. It seems that confinement prevents development of this strategy. Furthermore, the rats from the confinement group did not show any preference for a particular angle. The author supposed that a clockwise strategy is based on locomotor activity and that implementation of few seconds of delay is necessary to disrupt this motor-based strategy and allow animals to develop a spatial representation of the environment. Confinement intervals could range, in different versions of radial mazes, from seconds to minutes or tens of minutes (e.g. Dubreuil et al., 2003, Bolhuis et al., 1986). The original fully baited version of radial maze is designed to assess the working memory of animals. It is important to emphasize that the term ´working memory´ could be used with slightly different meanings for humans than for animals. Despite the differences, it seems that the animal concept of working memory is in accord with the human models in some respects (Keeler and Robbins, 2011). In a broader sense working memory in animals could be defined as a representation of object, stimulus or spatial location which is used to guide a behavior and is typically used within one testing session (Dudchenko, 2004). It could be problematic to distinguish working memory from other subtypes of short-term memory, but it is distinguishable from reference memory, a system of long-term memory. To test reference memory and working memory at the same time, a modified version of the radial maze was developed (Olton and Paras, 1979). This maze contains two sets of arms and only one of these sets is baited. The same arms contain food every day during the training. An animal has optimal performance when entering each of the baited arms only once on each trial and avoiding the unbaited set. The set which never contains the food represents the test of ´reference memory´ and entry to a never-baited arm is a reference memory error. The other arms containing the food constitute standard working memory test and repeated entry to one of these arms within one session is considered to be a working memory error.

In the context of neuropsychiatric disorders and their animal models, the radial maze has much attraction and is conventionally used to detect deficits in spatial working and reference memory in rats. A disadvantage of the test is that it may involve motor (or *praxis*) strategy of going successively from one arm to another, but this can be overcome by introducing a confinement interval between particular choices. Another issue could be the potential use of olfactory cues that indicate which arms have already been visited. Various methods to prevent the using of olfactory cues may be applied: it is possible to allow animals freely explore the maze before the test, thus the maze is saturated with aromatic cues; it is possible to clean the arms between the choices or to rotate them around the platform while the positions of the food remain the same (Sharma et al., 2010). The Olton radial maze has many advantages: it allows a study of several cognitive phenomena according to the experimental design that is used. The test is standardized and could be easily repeated in different laboratories. As mentioned before, spatial cognition is an intrinsic property of animal cognition and rodents could acquire the task quite easily. Moreover, the standard version of radial maze is appetitive and causes little stress to animals, except for the food restraint. The opportunity to separate working and reference memory and precisely quantify their deficits makes the radial maze powerful tool to model and study human neuropsychiatric disorders on their animal models, including schizophrenia, Alzheimer's disease, etc.

2.2.3 The Carousel maze

The Carousel maze (previously also termed active allothetic place avoidance (AAPA) or active place avoidance task (Stuchlik et al., 2004; Stuchlik and Vales, 2005; Vales et al., 2006, Stuchlik et al., 2009; Bubenikova-Valesova; 2008) or Room+/Arena- task (Weiserska et al., 2005; Kubik and Fenton 2005) is a variant of the place avoidance task (Bures et al., 1997, Bures et al., 1998; Fenton et al., 1998, Cimadevilla et al., 2000a,b,c; 2001a,b,c), in which a rodent (typically a rat, but the maze can be used with mice as well; Cimadevilla et al., 2001a) is placed on a smooth circular arena and required to avoid a directly imperceptible to-be-avoided sector. In the Carousel maze, the experimental arena slowly continuously rotates (1 rpm) in a lighted room and the to-be-avoided sector (60 deg) is defined in the fixed position in the coordinate frame of the room. Rats must therefore recognize the distal visual cues in the room, navigate according to them and ignore self-generated arena-based cues (urine, droppings, scent marks) which are dissociated from the to-be-avoided sector position by arena rotation. Animals also perceive arena rotation (which facilitates learning; Blahna et al., 2011) and have to find an appropriate active strategy moving constantly or in interrupted runs in the safe part of surface (hence active place avoidance). Behaviors in the Carousel maze can be evaluated by many parameters. The most frequently used measures include total distance traversed per session (as a measure of locomotion), number of errors (i.e., the number of entrances into the sector) and maximum time between two errors (maximum time avoided) showing cumulative performance within a session. The latency from the session start to the first error (latency to first error) shows the memory trace established on the previous day and thus can serve as a measure of retrieval of avoidance and may be suggestive of memory retrieval. There are additional measures which may characterize the track in a quantitative way (linearity of the trajectory, dwell-time in particular radial and annular zones, total number of shocks, percentage of time spent in the target quadrant and its counterparts and ´radial histogram´ measures). Many such parameters are provided by a formula for the place avoidance arena (Tracker, TrackAnalysis, Biosignal Group, USA).

2.2.3.1 Development of place avoidance tasks and Carousel maze

The original ´place avoidance´ tasks were developed in the late nineties (e.g. Bures et. al., 1997). The design of a ´dry-land´ spatial maze brought several major advantages:

1. It facilitated place-cell recordings (although the first, but very important paper on place cells´ behavior in a two-frame place avoidance task was published no earlier than 2010; Kelemen and Fenton, 2010).
2. It tested animal spatial learning and memory capabilities in a more natural environment than the Morris water maze, which later turned out to be a convenient tool in animal models of schizophrenia (Stuchlik et al., 2004; Stuchlik and Vales 2005, Vales et al., 2006; Bubenikova-Valesova et al., 2008, Vales et. al., 2010).
3. These tasks together with the selective usage of a constantly rotating arena and light/dark conditions allowed the definition of a to-be-avoided sector in the coordinate frames of either room or the arena (these two might be dissociated by slow arena rotation). This strongly advanced scientific views on the organization of information into the reference frames and the role of hippocampus (Fenton et al., 1998; Cimadevilla et al., 2001a) and ultimately to the discovery of a *´cognitive coordination´* function of the hippocampus (Wesierska et al., 2005). This showed that this *´frame-segregation´* function of the hippocampus is dissociable from the navigational function (Kubik and Fenton, 2005). Moreover, the aforementioned electro-physiological paper (Kelemen and Fenton, 2010) provided evidence for a neural substrate of cognitive control in this structure, showing that representations of the arena and room frames alternate in the hippocampus during solution of the two-frame place avoidance task requiring simultaneous avoidance of dissociated room and arena sectors. It is noteworthy that the Carousel maze was the task in which a blockade of maintenance phase of *long-term potentiation* (LTP) was found to erase a previously established memory trace as first (Pastalkova et al., 2006).
4. In particular, the Carousel maze has proved to be a suitable test of altered behavior in animal models of brain disorders, mainly schizophrenia (a pharmacological model induced by systemic treatment with a psychotomimetic MK-801, a non-competitive NMDA receptor antagonist) and has been used in several animal model studies todate (Stuchlik et al., 2004; Stuchlik and Vales, 2005; Vales et al., 2006, Bubenikova-Valesova et al., 2008, Stuchlik et al., 2009, Vales et al., 2010). Notably, the task was not found to be sensitive to an electrolytic lesion of the posterior parietal cortex (Svoboda et al., 2008), but is dependent on an intact retrosplenial cortex (RSC; Wesierska et al., 2009). More

specifically, the versions that involve conflict or motion of frames are impaired suggesting a role of the RSC in cognitive coordination.

2.2.3.2 Properties of the place avoidance and Carousel maze

It has been shown that rats learning the place avoidance tasks are capable of simultaneous and independent knowledge for arena- and room-frame memories (or representations; Fenton et al., 1998) and variants of the place avoidance tasks generally include those with no conflict in these two frames (e.g. both frames stable, or one artificially suppressed, see Wesierska et al., 2005) and modifications involving a conflict between frames. This is the case of the Carousel maze, where the arena and information based on its surface rotates, whilst the lighted room and to-be-avoided sector are stable. Hypothetically, a similar conflict of frames would occur in the avoidance of the to-be-avoided sector rotating together with the arena (defined in the arena frame) in the stable room. The ability to organize two dissociated references frames reflects a cognitive coordination function (see above). Passive versions of the task (where the animals do not have to actively move in order to solve it efficiently) are usually used with so-called *´pellet-retrieval´* (or pellet-chasing, Muller, 1996). This means that food-deprived avoiding rats are trained to collect small food pellets periodically dispersed onto random places of the arena floor from an overhead feeder. Contrary to passive versions, in the active versions of the task, such as the Carousel maze (active place avoidance), or a Carousel maze with shallow water suppressing the disturbing intra-maze cues (conflict between frames minimized), it is not necessary to motivate the animals to collect food, however, our experience suggests that random collecting for the scattered food during avoidance gives less variability in data and provides a sharper resolution for drug effects. However, it should be noted that this procedure failed to be useful for mice, which are usually tested on the arena covered with a grid.

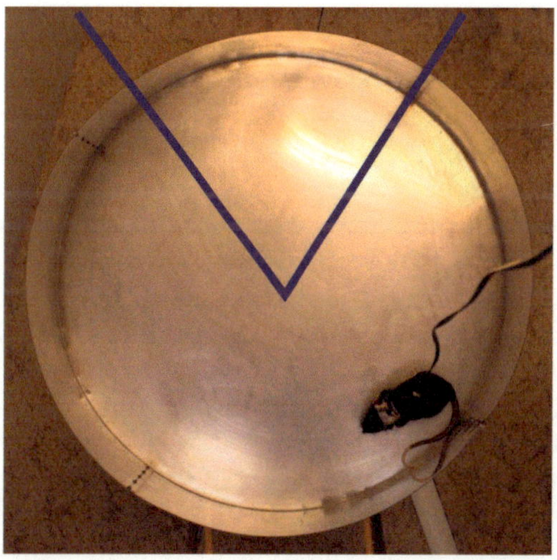

Fig. 1. A laboratory rat in the Carousel maze. The arena rotates and a to-be-avoided sector is defined in a particular part of the arena. The sector is unmarked (directly imperceptible), it is defined solely by the tracking program, it is delineated by the blue line in the figure.

The Carousel maze is a specific spatial learning task in several aspects. The sector is defined with respect to distal room cues, so the animals are required to use a purely allothetic (Mittelstaedt and Mittelstaedt, 1980) strategy for determining its position. The allothetic mode of information consists of distal orienting, mainly visual cues. It has been demonstrated that rats cannot acquire this task in darkness (unpublished results). The idiothetic mode of navigation (referring to the collection and integration of self-motion signals, (Mittelstaedt and Mittelstaedt, 1980, Mittelstaedt and Glasauer, 1991) and substratal exteroceptive cues such as scent marks which are normally crucial for learning on a dry arena; (Stuchlik et al., 2001; Stuchlik and Bures, 2002) are irrelevant and animals need to ignore them. Another feature of the task is that it requires an active approach for successful avoidance behavior. Passive strategies such as freezing or simple escape upon shock exposure represent an inefficient strategy, since arena rotation repeatedly transports the rat into the shock sector if the animal does not actively avoid it. The typical strategy to avoid punishment is to recognize the position of the shock sector and stay away from it by walking in a direction opposite to arena rotation. Another advantage of the task is that it is acquired very rapidly (depending on the variant, even faster than in the Morris water maze or radial maze). It is therefore possible to assess even short-term changes in performance of animals, e.g. during the oestrous cycle (Cimadevilla et al., 2000b). Since the Carousel maze is a dry-arena task, it does not require swimming and thus can be applied to as young as weanling rats (Cimadevilla et al., 2001b).

Very straightforward support for the usage of the Carousel maze and place avoidance tasks in general in the research of animal models comes from a study of Abdel Baki et al., 2009. Instead of using single-condition avoidance, the authors designed a hierarchy of place avoidance tasks consisting of passive and active versions with incrementally increasing demand for the segregation of frames and showed that this battery is capable of discriminating between mild and moderate brain injury (Abdel Baki et al., 2009). Indeed, for use in animal models, (which is favorable, the test is rapidly acquired by intact rats; Stuchlik et al.,. 2004) it should be emphasized that it is preferable to use more conditions of the place avoidance with different requirements for frame segregation, either successively as in lesion and neurodevelopmental models; (Abdel Baki et al., 2009; Stuchlik et al., 2011) or in different animals (for drug treatments). This allows for interpretation of data in terms of the cognitive coordination hypothesis (see above) rather than mere acquisition of room-based place avoidance on the rotating arena. We propose that pure acquisition of the Carousel maze task such as used in Stuchlik et al., 2004; Vales et al., 2006; and Stuchlik et al., 2009 represents a mixture of contribution in *allothetic* learning, skill learning (Dockery and Weiserska, 2010) and coordination of arena and room frames (Wesierska et al., 2005, Kubik and Fenton, 2005, Kubik et al., 2006). It is recommended to pursue a pre-exposure (*habituation*) to the environment. Some form of pre-training prior to manipulations should be also considered (Stuchlik and Vales, 2005; Vales and Stuchlik, 2005). Performance in the Carousel maze was demonstrated to be overtly impaired also by NMDA-induced lesion of the dorsal hippocampus as a model of excitotoxic damage to the brain (Rambousek et al., 2011), such as in the case of ischemia or stroke. In some cases, however, the locomotor activity in the Carousel maze was found to be altered by lower doses of drugs than spatial avoidance parameters (Stuchlik et al., 2007b). Therefore, it is favorable to design tests without locomotor components, such as spatially-driven operant tasks, described in the following chapter.

2.2.4 Spatial operant tasks using the computer screen and a Skinner box

Rodent spatial cognition is conventionally investigated mainly by tasks in which animals actively move in the environment (e.g. Morris, 1981). Disrupted performance in this case may therefore be caused by deficits in recognizing subject's own position and/or planning and executing goal-directed movements. Attempts have been made to minimize the influence of locomotor components, while extracting recognition components of animal behavior. In experiments by Klement and Bures (2000) rats were passively transported onto a rotating arena through an environment. They were trained to recognize a specific position by reinforcing lever presses at that location. Pastalkova et al. (2003) studied rats watching a rotating scene. These animals were trained to respond when the scene was within a particular sector by reinforcing lever presses while the object was there.

Scientists also developed a behavioral test in which rats observe distant objects on a computer screen, and discriminate their positions by responding to them with a lever press (Nekovarova and Klement, 2006, Klement et al., 2008; Nekovarova et al., 2009; Klement et al., 2010.). Food-deprived rats were placed in a modified Skinner box with an open front wall allowing them to view the screen. The operant chamber was placed in front of a computer screen where the visual stimuli were presented. The rats were trained to press a lever according to these stimuli. The operant responses were rewarded when a particular stimulus or configuration was displayed. We used this experimental apparatus for tasks measuring various types of cognition, i.e., brightness discrimination, object discrimination, and position-discrimination. In the position-discrimination task, rats are trained to press a lever when a stationary object was displayed in a particular position, or when a moving object was passing through a particular region. Animals increased number of responses before the object entered the rewarded area. This suggests these animals recognized the position of the virtual object moving on the computer screen by estimating distance between the object and the rewarded position (Klement et al., 2010).

Other rewarding protocols were also explored in these spatio-operant tests. In other experiments (Nekovarova and Bures, 2006; Nekovarova et. al., 2006), the apparatus consisted of an animal chamber with transparent front wall with four nosing holes organized in the rectangle matrix, arms with water dippers, a water reservoir and a computer monitor. The front wall faced a computer monitor serving to present visual stimuli. The nosing holes in the front wall were equipped by photoelectric devices registering a nose poke in a particular nosing hole. Two dippers (capacity 0.15 ml) were movable before the front wall. They served to deliver the reward to the animal. They could be raised by electric motors from the water reservoir placed below the box to the level of the particular nosing holes as a result of the animal's correct responses. A transparent sliding barrier, parallel to the front wall, could be closed and prevent access to the nosing holes. The computer registered nose-poking, activated electric motors operating the barrier and the dippers, and displayed graphics on the monitor screen. Initially, water-deprived rats were used and water was presented as a reward. The advantage of this method is the urgency. Rats are highly motivated to respond. However, it is quite difficult to maintain motivation of laboratory animals. Later, a sugar solution was used. Thus, it was not necessary to maintain the rats as water-deprived (which could be quite stressful) and the animals are motivated to respond during the whole day-session. This experimental design was used for the study of higher cognitive functions in rats. We studied their ability to decode abstract visual stimuli containing the spatial (configuration) information. Two types of stimuli were presented: 1) Spatial stimuli - They were designed as a simple representation (map) of the real response space (configuration of nosing holes). These stimuli contained configuration information. 2) Non-spatial stimuli – These were simple geometrical patterns without any implicit configuration information. Every picture was connected to a single nosing hole. It was shown that spatial stimuli could be used more effectively than non-spatial stimuli. This experimental apparatus had several advantages. Since exploration is natural behavior for rats, the nose-poking was easier for rats as an operant response than lever-pressing. Another advantage was the opportunity to present wide range of stimuli on the computer screen.

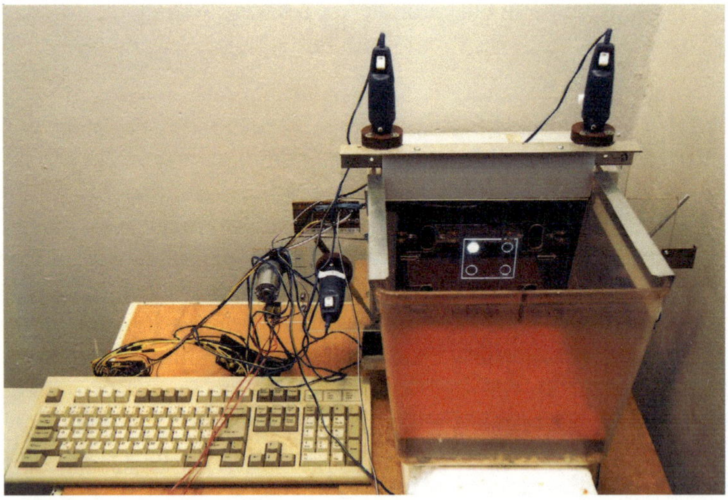

Fig. 2. A photograph of the spatio-operant task designed for studying rats' ability to discriminate position or movement of an object presented on a computer screen. During the test, an animal is placed in the operant box and responds to stimuli projected on the computer monitor with a lever press or nose-poking.

In order to test the usability of this task for pharmacological and animal model research, Levcik examined the effect of systemic injection of MK-801, (RS)-2-chloro-5-hydroxyphenylglycine (CHPG, an mGluR5-agonist), and co-administration of both substances on the cognitive performance of rats in this novel spatial task (Levcik et al., 2010). Food-restrained rats were trained to press a lever when an object (white rectangle) moving from one side of the screen to the other was in the particular ´rewarded area´. After the rats had reached the point of asymptotic performance, the effect of MK-801 and CHPG on spatial cognition was tested. Whereas intact rats showed increased frequency before the object entered into the rewarded area, MK-801 (0.1 mg/kg, i.p.) impaired the ability of animals to recognize the position of the distant objects on the screen, without affecting motor activity. Administration of CHPG (0.1 mg/kg, i.p.) did not elicit an effect on either the cognitive or motor component of the performance. Treatment with CHPG reduced MK-801-induced impairment of performance of the task, consistent with findings in other laboratories.

These observations suggest that the test provides a novel tool suitable for evaluating disturbances of spatial cognition in animal models of CNS disorders. The major benefit of this novel task, e.g. in comparison with MWM and radial maze, is the ability to dissect between cognitive and motor components of animal behavior, which is advantageous particularly in pharmacological research, because many drugs also affect locomotor functions besides learning and cognitive processes. A disadvantage of this method is the relatively long training time compared to other tasks. In operant response to spatial cues rats also tend to use spatial and temporal strategies; rats may use both of them in many versions of these operant tasks. Therefore, it is important to design these tasks in a way that allows a distinction between these strategies. Use of large computer LCD screens provides better control of the shapes of objects, their positions, velocity, and trajectories, as well as the precise timing of experiments. These manipulations may be difficult with physical objects. Moreover, these ´virtual reality´ tasks are applicable also to primates and humans (Nekovarova et al., 2009), i.e. they are fully translational. This allows better understanding of the difference in neuronal mechanisms and functions across species, and, thus, better prediction of the ability of novel drugs to ameliorate cognitive impairments in human patients.

2.2.5 Enemy avoidance task

The enemy avoidance task in rats was first introduced by Telensky (2009) and the task can be defined as avoidance of a moving conspecific (Telensky et al., 2009) or a mobile object (Telensky et al., 2011). Quite different from the classic avoidance that a rodent would exert facing a real predator or cat odor, the avoidance behavior is reinforced by completely artificial, but well-controlled and reproducible aversive stimulus - electric footshock.

There is an imperceptible zone surrounding the moving stimulus, upon entering the tested subject rat receives a mild footshock and a normal rat eventually learns to avoid such a stimulus with a rapid escape reaction but no signs distress (it still retains foraging for randomly scattered food). It should be kept in mind when interpreting data from this model that it was not designed to reproduce natural defensive behaviors of rats, but developed in the context of the concept of multiple and mutually independent reference frames, such as the dissociated arena and room reference frames in the Carousel maze (see above). In the Carousel maze, two-frame place avoidance and place avoidance tasks in general, brain representations have been studied for coordination function, i.e. segregation and organization of dissociated reference frames (Wesierska et al., 2005, Kubik and Fenton, 2005; Kelemen and Fenton, 2010). An intriguing hypothesis was proposed that such a reference frame could be represented by a moving entity, such as some animal or a thing. The tests were also intended to allow studying physiological substrate of these functions (such as representation of a moving stimulus or even a frame of reference) using lesion, inactivation and electrophysiological measurements. Such an approach was used in the second study, exploiting a moving programmable robot, which showed that avoidance of a moving robot required the hippocampus but avoidance of a stable robot did not.

The first study (Telensky et al., 2009) used a conspecific as the moving object. A laboratory rat (subject) was trained to avoid another rat (enemy), while searching for small pasta pellets dispensed onto an experimental arena. Whenever the distance between the two animals dropped bellow 25cm, the subject obtained a mild electric footshock. This study showed that rats are capable of avoiding another rat while exploring an environment, suggesting that rat are able to represent moving entities. It should be noted that the learning of this task was relatively slow and required some period of immobilization (with a cage) of the enemy.

However, the predictability of the enemy rat's movement is obviously slow; moreover rats are known to posses agonistic interactions. The second study (Telensky et al., 2011), thus, used a small mobile robot, which could serve as the center of a to-be-avoided zone in two basic configurations - stable and mobile. In the moving-object configuration, the robot traversed the arena linearly and upon touching the wall it turned a random angle and started to traverse the arena straight again. In the stable-object version, it remained stable and was only moved randomly at longer intervals to prevent place learning. Interestingly, functional inactivation of the dorsal hippocampus with stereotaxic microinjection of teterodotoxin (TTX), sodium channel blocker, which causes cessation of neuronal firing (Zhuravin and Bures, 1991; Klement et al., 2005) disrupted avoidance of the moving but not the stable robot.

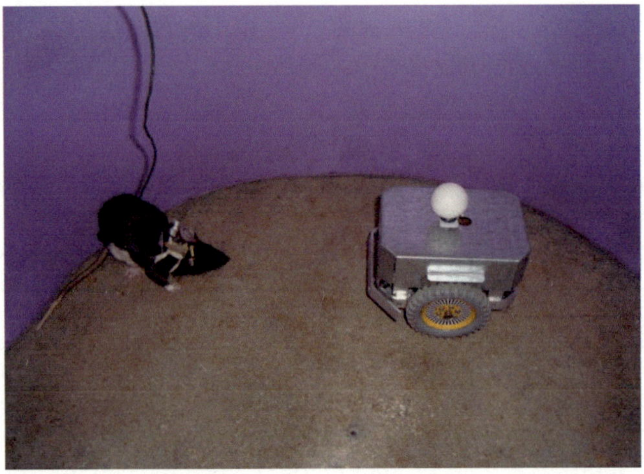

Fig. 3. A laboratory rat solving the Enemy avoidance task. Photograph: Jan Svoboda. Rats foraging for small pasta pellets dropped on the arena floor from an overhead feeder learned to avoid both a stable and randomly moving robot. Nonetheless, navigation with respect to moving robot required an intact hippocampus (Telensky et al., 2011), but avoidance of the stable robot did not. (c) Jan Svoboda

Another interesting test similar to this task but appetitive in nature was proposed in 2008 (Ho et al., 2008), when the authors used a small moving toy car and animals were trained to approach the moving car and this approach was rewarded by intra-cranial stimulation (ICS) (Olds and Milner, 1957; Ho et al., 2008). Activity of hippocampal place-cells was measured. The car-dependent navigation task involved a car inside the arena, and animals obtained a brain reward if it approached and came within 20 cm of the car. In car-independent navigation, the rats were rewarded for traveling 150cm regardless of relation to the car. Place fields were remapped more frequently in the car-dependent than car-independent tasks. Place cell activity in both conditions showed moderate tuning to the movement parameters of the rats and car, and the distance between the car and rats. Place-cell tuning to the movement variables of the car was more specific in the version with the car than without the car. The coding of movement variables of the car by the place-cell activity was larger in the car-dependent than car-independent task. This intriguing study showed that activity of hippocampal place cells may represent not only an animal's own location but also the movement parameters of another moving object if it is associated with a reward. The study also suggests a neural correlate of representation of a moving object in the activity of place cells localized to the hippocampus. The recent study (Telensky et al., 2011) supports findings of the study by Ho et al. and these findings showed the requirement of functional hippocampal integrity for such a representation of a moving object, defined here in the aversive terms. These results also seem to extend Cognitive Map Theory of the hippocampus function (O'Keefe and Nadel, 1978) showing that visibility is not the sole decisive factor for hippocampus-dependence of the task and that stability and/or motion of object must be considered as well. This view has a close analogy with a proposed role of hippocampus in the *'automatic recording of attended experience'* (Morris and Frey, 1997). Continuous updating of the dynamically changing position of a moving object may thus represent such a phenomenon. Studies aimed at these abilities are required for pre-clinical research, because in many brain disorders, such information flow and working memory capabilities strongly decline, such as in psychoses or dementias. However, it must be noted that the translational potential of the test is yet unexplored. For use in humans the test has to be made appetitive and simplified to provide easy administration and evaluation. This is in the plans of our laboratory.

3. Conclusion

Pre-clinical research into animal models of CNS disorders require appropriate behavioral tests for detection of outcomes of brain manipulation pursued in the model. This work has surveyed some of the classically used tests such as radial or Morris water mazes and introduced several novel tests, which have the potential to be used in animal model research due to the specific functions they examine (*place navigation, cognitive coordination, continuous updating of position of a moving stimulus*). Application of these tasks in the research of animal models of CNS disorders and accompanying cognitive and information-processing deficits is still a work in progress. Experiments are being performed with moving stimuli in animal models of cognitive deficit and in animal models of schizophrenia-like behaviors induced by low dose MK-801, a high-affinity non-competitive NMDA receptor antagonist. The hippocampus requirement of these tasks (Wesierska et al., 2005; Kubik and Fenton, 2005, Telensky et al., 2011) and their aim at spatial navigation (as a model of declarative memory) and other higher cognitive functions (impaired in many neuropsychiatric diseases) suggest that they might become a powerful tool in pre-clinical research oriented toward animal models and the discovery of drugs aimed at cognitive functions.

4. Acknowledgment

The authors express gratitude to Dr. Jan Bures for critical opinions and scientific inspiration. Thanks belong also to Peter M. Luketic for the language review of the draft and to all members of the laboratory for their support. This study was supported by GACR grants P303/10/J032 and 309/09/0286, GACR Center of Excellence P304/12/G069 and by AV0Z50110509. All authors were also supported by AV0Z50110509

5. References

Abdel Baki, S.G., Kao, H.Y., Kelemen, E., Fenton, A.A., Bergold, P.J. (2009). A hierarchy of neurobehavioral tasks discriminates between mild and moderate brain injury in rats. Brain Research, Vol. 1280, pp. 98-106, ISSN 0006-8993

Adler, L.E., Pachtman, E., Franks, R.D., Pecevich, M., Waldo, M.C., Freedman, R. (1982). Neurophysiological evidence for a defect in neuronal mechanisms involved in sensory gating in schizophrenia. Biological Psychiatry. Vol. 17, No. 6, pp. 639-654, ISSN 0006-3223

Adler, L.E., Rose, G., Freedman, R. (1986). Neurophysiological studies of sensory gating in rats: effects of amphetamine, phencyclidine, and haloperidol. Biological Psychiatry. Vol. 21, No. 8-9, pp. 787-98, ISSN 0006-3223

Ammassari-Teule, M., Caprioli, A. (1985). Spatial learning and memory, maze running strategies and cholinergic mechanisms in two inbred strains of mice. Behavioral Brain Research, Vol.17, No. 1, pp. 9-16, ISSN 0166-4328

Arnt, J., Skarsfeldt, T., Hyttel, J. (1997). Differentiation of classical and novel antipsychotics using animal models. International Clinical Psychopharmacology, Vol. 12, Suppl 1, pp. S9-S17, ISSN 1473-5857

Auclair, A.L., Kleven, M.S., Besnard, J., Depoortère, R., Newman-Tancredi, A. (2006). Actions of novel antipsychotic agents on apomorphine-induced PPI disruption: influence of combined serotonin 5-HT1A receptor activation and dopamine D2 receptor blockade. Neuropsychopharmacology,, Vol. 31, No. 9, pp. 1900-1909, ISSN 0893-133X

Baker, N.J., Staunton, M., Adler, L.E., Gerhardt, G.A., Drebing, C., Waldo, M., Nagamoto, H., Freedman, R. (1990). Sensory gating deficits in psychiatric inpatients: relation to catecholamine metabolites in different diagnostic groups. Biological Psychiatry, Vol. 27, No. 5, pp.519-528, ISSN 0006-3223

Bakshi, V.P., Swerdlow, N.R., Braff, D.L., Geyer, M.A. (1998). Reversal of isolation rearing-induced deficits in prepulse inhibition by Seroquel and olanzapine. Biological Psychiatry. Vol. 43, No. 6, pp. 436-445, ISSN 0006-3223

Beiko, J., Candusso, L., Cain, D.P. (1997). The effect of nonspatial water maze pretraining in rats subjected to serotonin depletion and muscarinic receptor antagonism: a detailed behavioural assessment of spatial performance. Behavioral Brain Research, Vol. 88, No. 2, pp. 201-211, ISSN 0166-4328

Benhamou, S. (1997). Path integration by swimming rats. Animal Behaviour, Vol. 54, No. 2, pp. 321-327, ISSN: 0003-3472

Blahna, K., Svoboda, J., Telensky, P., Klement, D. (2011). Inertial stimuli generated by arena rotation are important for acquisition of the active place avoidance task. Behavioral Brain Research, Vol. 216, No. 1, pp. 207-213, ISSN 0166-4328

Bolhuis, J.J., Bijlsma, S., Ansmink, P. (1986). Exponential decay of spatial memory of rats in a radial maze. Behavioral and Neural Biology, Vol. 46, No. 2, pp. 115-122, ISSN 0163-1047

Braff, D.L., Geyer, M.A. (1990). Sensorimotor gating and schizophrenia. Human and animal model studies. Archives of General Psychiatry, Vol. 47, No. 2, pp. 181-188, ISSN 0003-990x

Braff, D.L., Grillon, C., Geyer, M.A. (1992). Gating and habituation of the startle reflex in schizophrenic patients. Archives of General Psychiatry, Vol. 49, No. 3, pp. 206-215, ISSN 0003-990x

Broadbent, N.J., Squire, L.R., Clark, R.E. (2006). Reversible hippocampal lesions disrupt water maze performance during both recent and remote memory tests. Learning and Memory, Vol. 13, pp. 187–191, ISSN 1072-0502

Bubeníková, V., Votava, M., Horácek, J., Pálenícek, T. (2005a). Relation of sex and estrous phase to deficits in prepulse inhibition of the startle response induced by ecstasy (MDMA). Behavioural Pharmacology, Vol. 16, No. 2, pp. 127-130, ISSN 0955-8810

Bubeníková, V., Votava, M., Horácek, J., Pálenícek, T., Dockery, C. (2005b). The effect of zotepine, risperidone, clozapine and olanzapine on MK-801-disrupted sensorimotor gating. Pharmacology, Biochemistry and Behavior, Vol. 80, No. 4, pp. 591-596, ISSN 0091-3057

Bubeníková-Valesová, V., Votava, M., Pálenícek, T., Horácek, J. (2007). The opposite effect of a low and a high dose of serotonin-1A agonist on behavior induced by MK-801. Neuropharmacology, Vol. 52, No. 4, pp. 1071-1078, ISSN 0028-3908

Bubenikova-Valesova, V., Stuchlik, A., Svoboda, J., Bures, J., Vales, K. (2008a). Risperidone and ritanserin but not haloperidol block effect of dizocilpine on the active allothetic place avoidance task. Proceedings of the National Academy of Sciences, USA, Vol. 105, No. 3, pp. 1061-1066, ISSN 0027-8424

Bubeníková-Valesová, V., Horácek, J., Vrajová, M., Höschl, C. (2008b). Models of schizophrenia in humans and animals based on inhibition of NMDA receptors. Neuroscience and Biobehavioral Reviews, Vol. 32, No. 5, pp. 1014-1023, ISSN 0149-7634

Bures, J., Fenton, A.A., Kaminsky, Y., Zinyuk, L. (1997). Place cells and place navigation. Proceedings of the National Academy of Sciences, USA, Vol. 94, No. 1, pp. 343-350, ISSN 0027-8424

Bures, J., Fenton, A.A., Kaminsky, Y., Wesierska, M., Zahalka, A. (1998). Rodent navigation after dissociation of the allocentric and idiothetic representations of space. Neuropharmacology, Vol.37, No. 4-5, pp. 689-699,

Buresová, O., Bures, J. (1982). Radial maze as a tool for assessing the effect of drugs on the working memory of rats. Psychopharmacology, Vol. 77, No. 3, pp. 268-271, ISSN 0033-3158

Buresová, O., Bures, J., Oitzl, M.S., Zahálka, A. (1985a). Radial maze in the water tank: an aversively motivated spatial working memory task. Physiology and Behavior, Vol. 34, No. 6, pp. 1003-1005, ISSN 0031-9384

Buresová, O., Krekule, I., Zahálka, A., Bures, J. (1985b). On-demand platform improves accuracy of the Morris water maze procedure. Journal of Neuroscience Methods, Vol. 15, No. 1, pp. 63-72, ISSN 0165-0270

Cain, D.P., Saucier, D., Boon, F. (1997a). Testing hypotheses of spatial learning: the role of NMDA receptors and NMDA-mediated long-term potentiation. Behavioral Brain Research, Vol. 84, No. 1-2, pp. 179-193, ISSN 0166-4328

Cain, D.P. (1997b). Prior non-spatial pretraining eliminates sensorimotor disturbances and impairments in water maze learning caused by diazepam. Psychopharmacology, Vol. 130, No. 4, pp. 313-319, ISSN 0033-3158

Castagné, V., Moser, P.C., Porsolt, R.D. (2009). Preclinical behavioral models for predicting antipsychotic activity. Advances in Pharmacology, Vol. 57, pp. 381-418, ISSN 1054-3589

Castellanos, F.X., Fine, E.J., Kaysen, D., Marsh, W.L., Rapoport, J.L., Hallett, M. (1996). Sensorimotor gating in boys with Tourette's syndrome and ADHD: preliminary results. Biological Psychiatry, Vol. 39, No. 1, pp. 33-41, ISSN 0006-3223

Cimadevilla, J.M., Kaminsky, Y., Fenton, A., Bures, J. (2000a). Passive and active place avoidance as a tool of spatial memory research in rats. Journal of Neuroscience Methods, Vol. 102, No. 2, pp. 155-164, ISSN 0165-0270

Cimadevilla, J.M., Fenton, A.A., Bures, J. (2000b). Continuous place avoidance task reveals differences in spatial navigation in male and female rats. Behavioral Brain Research, Vol. 107, No. 1-2, pp. 161-169, ISSN 0166-4328

Cimadevilla, J.M., Fenton, A.A., Bures, J. (2000c). Functional inactivation of dorsal hippocampus impairs active place avoidance in rats. Neuroscience Letters, Vol. 285, No. 1, pp. 53-56, ISSN 0304-3940

Cimadevilla, J.M., Fenton, A.A., Bures, J. (2001a). New spatial cognition tests for mice: passive place avoidance on stable and active place avoidance on rotating arenas. Brain Research Bulletin, Vol. 54, No. 5, pp. 559-563, ISSN: 0361-9230

Cimadevilla, J.M., Fenton, A.A., Bures, J. (2001b). Transient sex differences in the between-sessions but not in the within-session memory underlying an active place avoidance task in weanling rats. Behavioral Neuroscience, Vol. 115, No. 3, pp. 695-703, ISSN 0735-7044

Cimadevilla, J.M., Wesierska, M., Fenton, A.A., Bures, J. (2001c). Inactivating one hippocampus impairs avoidance of a stable room-defined place during dissociation of arena cues from room cues by rotation of the arena. Proceedings of the National Academy of Sciences, USA, Vol. 98, No. 6, pp. 3531-3536, ISSN 0027-8424

Clark, R.E., Martin, S.J. (2005a). Interrogating rodents regarding their object and spatial memory. Current Opinion in Neurobiology, Vol. 15, No. 5, pp. 593-598, ISSN 0959-4388

Clark, R.E., Broadbent, N.J., Squire, L.R. (2005b). Hippocampus and remote spatial memory in rats. Hippocampus, Vol. 15, pp. 260–272, ISSN 1050-9631

Conzelmann, A., Pauli, P., Mucha, R.F., Jacob, C.P., Gerdes, A.B., Romanos, J., Bähne, C.G., Heine, M., Boreatti-Hümmer, A., Alpers, G.W., Fallgatter, A.J., Warnke, A., Lesch, K.P., Weyers, P. (2010). Early attentional deficits in an attention-to-prepulse paradigm in ADHD adults. J Abnorm Psychol. Vol. 119, No. 3, pp. 594-603, ISSN 1050-9631

Cook, R.G., Brown, M.F., Riley, D.A. (1985). Flexible memory processing by rats: use of prospective and retrospective information in the radial maze. Journal of Experimental Psychology: Animal Behavior Processes, Vol. 11, No. 3, pp. 453-469, ISSN 0097-7403

de Bruin, N.M., Ellenbroek, B.A., Cools, A.R., Coenen, A.M., van Luijtelaar, E.L. (1999). Differential effects of ketamine on gating of auditory evoked potentials and prepulse inhibition in rats. Psychopharmacology, Vol. 142, No. 1, pp. 9-17, ISSN 0033-3158

D'Hooge, R., De Deyn, P.P. (2001). Applications of the Morris water maze in the study of learning and memory. Brain Research Reviews, Vol. 36, No. 1, pp. 60-90, ISSN 0165-0173

Dockery, C.A., Wesierska, M.J. (2010). A spatial paradigm, the allothetic place avoidance alternation task, for testing visuospatial working memory and skill learning in rats. Journal of Neuroscience Methods, Vol. 191, No. 2, pp. 215-221, ISSN 0165-0270

Dubreuil, D., Tixier, C., Dutrieux, G., Edeline, J.M. (2003). Does the radial arm maze necessarily test spatial memory? Neurobiology of Learning and Memory, Vol. 79, No. 1, pp. 109-117, ISSN 1074-7427

Dudchenko, P.A. (2004). An overview of the tasks used to test working memory in rodents. Neuroscience and Biobehavioral Reviews, Vol. 28, No. 7, pp. 699-709,

Dvorkin, A., Culver, K.E., Waxman, D., Szechtman, H., Kolb, B. (2008). Effects of hypophysectomy on compulsive checking and cortical dendrites in an animal model of obsessive-compulsive disorder. Behavioural Pharmacology, Vol. 19, No. 4, pp. 271-283, ISSN 0955-8810

Dvorkin, A., Silva, C., McMurran, T., Bisnaire, L., Foster, J., Szechtman, H. (2010). Features of compulsive checking behavior mediated by nucleus accumbens and orbital frontal cortex. European Journal of Neuroscience, Vol. 32, No. 9, pp. 1552-1563, online ISSN 1460-9568

Ellenbroek, B.A., Cools, A.R. (1990). Animal models with construct validity for schizophrenia. Behavioural Pharmacology, Vol. 1, No. 6, pp. 469-490, ISSN 0955-8810

Ellenbroek, B.A., van den Kroonenberg, P.T., Cools, A.R. (1998). The effects of an early stressful life event on sensorimotor gating in adult rats. Schizophrenia Research, Vol. 30, No. 3, pp. 251-260, ISSN 0920-9964

Ellenbroek, B.A., Cools, A.R. (2000). The long-term effects of maternal deprivation depend on the genetic background. Neuropsychopharmacology,, Vol. 23, No. 1, pp. 99-106, ISSN 0893-133X

Fenton, A.A., Wesierska, M., Kaminsky, Y., Bures, J. (1998). Both here and there: simultaneous expression of autonomous spatial memories in rats. Proceedings of the National Academy of Sciences, USA, Vol. 95, No. 19, pp. 11493-11498, ISSN 0027-8424

Franks, R.D., Adler, L.E., Waldo, M.C., Alpert, J., Freedman, R. (1983). Neurophysiological studies of sensory gating in mania: comparison with schizophrenia. Biological Psychiatry, Vol. 18, No. 9, pp. 989-1005, ISSN 0006-3223

Garthe, A., Behr, J., Kempermann, G. (2009). Adult-generated hippocampal neurons allow the flexible use of spatially precise learning strategies. PLoS ONE, Vol. 4, No. 5, pp. e5464, EISSN 1932-6203

Geyer, M.A., Wilkinson, L.S., Humby, T., Robbins, T.W. (1993). Isolation rearing of rats produces a deficit in prepulse inhibition of acoustic startle similar to that in schizophrenia. Biological Psychiatry, Vol. 34, No. 6, pp. 361-372, ISSN 0006-3223

Geyer, M.A., McIlwain, K.L., Paylor, R.(2002). Mouse genetic models for prepulse inhibition: an early review. Molecular Psychiatry, Vol. 7, No. 10, pp. 1039-1053, ISSN 1359-4184

Geyer, M.A. (2008). Developing translational animal models for symptoms of schizophrenia or bipolar mania. Neurotoxicity Research, Vol. 14, No. 1, pp. 71-78, ISSN 1029-8428

Giakoumaki, S.G., Roussos, P., Rogdaki, M., Karli, C., Bitsios, P., Frangou, S. (2007). Evidence of disrupted prepulse inhibition in unaffected siblings of bipolar disorder patients. Biological Psychiatry, Vol. 62, No. 12, pp. 1418-1422, ISSN 0006-3223

Hafting, T., Fyhn, M., Molden, S., Moser, M.B., Moser, EI. (2005). Microstructure of a spatial map in the entorhinal cortex. Nature, Vol. 436, No. 7052, pp. 801-806, ISSN 0028-0836

Hejl, A.M., Glenthøj, B., Mackeprang, T., Hemmingsen, R., Waldemar, G. (2004). Prepulse inhibition in patients with Alzheimer's disease. Neurobiology of Aging, Vol. 25, No. 8, pp. 1045-1050, ISSN 0197-4580

Ho, S.A., Hori, E., Kobayashi, T., Umeno, K., Tran, A.H., Ono, T., Nishijo, H.(2008). Hippocampal place cell activity during chasing of a moving object associated with reward in rats. Neuroscience, Vol. 157, No. 1, pp. 254-270, ISSN 0306-4522

Hoenig, K., Hochrein, A., Quednow, B.B., Maier, W., Wagner, M. (2005). Impaired prepulse inhibition of acoustic startle in obsessive-compulsive disorder. Biological Psychiatry, Vol. 57, No. 10, pp. 1153-1158, ISSN 0006-3223

Hok, V., Save, E., Lenck-Santini, P.P., Poucet, B. (2005). Coding for spatial goals in the prelimbic/infralimbic area of the rat frontal cortex. Proceedings of the National Academy of Sciences, USA, Vol. 102, No. 12, pp. 4602-4607, ISSN 0027-8424

Hok, V., Lenck-Santini, P.P., Roux, S., Save, E., Muller, R.U., Poucet, B. (2007). Goal-related activity in hippocampal place cells. Journal of Neuroscience, Vol. 27, No. 3, pp. 472-482, ISSN 0270-6474

Hölscher, C. (1999). Stress impairs performance in spatial water maze learning tasks. Behavioral Brain Research, Vol. 100, No. 1-2, pp. 225-235, ISSN 0166-4328

Hort, J., Laczó, J., Vyhnálek, M., Bojar, M., Bures, J., Vlcek, K. (2007). Spatial navigation deficit in amnestic mild cognitive impairment. Proceedings of the National Academy of Sciences, USA, Vol. 104, No. 10, pp. 4042-4047, ISSN 0027-8424

Jones, C.K., Shannon, H.E. (2000). Muscarinic cholinergic modulation of prepulse inhibition of the acoustic startle reflex. Journal of Pharmacology and Experimental Therapeutics, Vol. 294, No. 3, pp. 1017-1023, ISSN 0022-3565

Keeler, J.F., Robbins, T.W. (2011). Translating cognition from animals to humans. Biochemical Pharmacology, Vol. 81, No. 12, pp. 1356-1366,

Kelemen, E., Fenton, A.A. (2010). Dynamic grouping of hippocampal neural activity during cognitive control of two spatial frames. PLoS Biology, Vol. 8, No. 6, pp. e1000403, ISSN-1544-9173

Klement, D., Bures, J. (2000). Place recognition monitored by location-driven operant responding during passive transport of the rat over a circular trajectory. Proceedings of the National Academy of Sciences, USA, Vol. 97, No. 6, pp. 2946-2951, ISSN 0027-8424

Klement D, Past'alková E, Fenton AA. (2005). Tetrodotoxin infusions into the dorsal hippocampus block non-locomotor place recognition. Hippocampus, Vol. 15, No. 4, pp. 460-471, ISSN 1050-9631

Klement, D., Blahna, K., Nekovárová, T. (2008). Novel behavioral tasks for studying spatial cognition in rats. Physiological Research, Vol.57, Suppl 3, pp. S161-S165, ISSN 0862-8408

Klement, D., Levcik, D., Duskova, L., Nekovarova, T. (2010). Spatial task for rats testing position recognition of an object displayed on a computer screen. Behavioral Brain Research, Vol. 207, No. 2, pp. 480-489, ISSN 0166-4328

Kubík, S., Fenton, A.A. (2005). Behavioral evidence that segregation and representation are dissociable hippocampal functions. Journal of Neuroscience, Vol. 25, No. 40, pp. 9205-9212, ISSN 0270-6474

Kubík, S., Stuchlík, A., Fenton, A.A. (2006). Evidence for hippocampal role in place avoidance other than merely memory storage. Physiological Research, Vol. 55, No. 4, pp. 445-452, ISSN 0862-8408

Kubik, S., Miyashita, T., Guzowski, J.F. (2007). Using immediate-early genes to map hippocampal subregional functions. Learning and Memory, Vol. 14, No. 11. pp. 758-770, ISSN 1072-0502

Le Pen, G., Moreau, J.L. (2002). Disruption of prepulse inhibition of startle reflex in a neurodevelopmental model of schizophrenia: reversal by clozapine, olanzapine and risperidone but not by haloperidol. Neuropsychopharmacology, Vol. 27, No. 1, pp. 1-11, ISSN 0028-3908

Levcik, D., Klement, D., Vales, K., Nekovarova, T., Stuchlik, A. (2010). Antagonist of NMDA receptors MK-801 disrupts recognition of the position of a distant object. Psychiatrie, Vol. 14, No. 2, pp. 15-18, ISSN 1211-7579

Lever, C., Burton, S., Jeewajee, A., O'Keefe, J., Burgess, N. (2009). Boundary vector cells in the subiculum of the hippocampal formation. Journal of Neuroscience, Vol. 29, No. 31, pp. 9771-9777, ISSN 0270-6474

Maguire, E.A., Nannery, R., Spiers, H.J. (2006). Navigation around London by a taxi driver with bilateral hippocampal lesions. Brain, Vol. 129, No. Pt 11, pp. 2894-2907, ISSN 0006-8950

Mansbach, R.S., Geyer, M.A., Braff, D.L. (1988). Dopaminergic stimulation disrupts sensorimotor gating in the rat. Psychopharmacology, Vol. 94, No. 4, pp. 507-514, ISSN 0033-3158

Mansbach, R.S., Geyer, M.A. (1989). Effects of phencyclidine and phencyclidine biologs on sensorimotor gating in the rat. Neuropsychopharmacology, Vol. 2, No. 4, pp.299-308, ISSN 0893-133X

Markowska, A.L., Long, J.M., Johnson, C.T., Olton, D.S. (1993). Variable-interval probe test as a tool for repeated measurements of spatial memory in the water maze. Behavioral Neuroscience. Vol. 107, No. 4, pp. 627-632, ISSN 0735-7044

Martin, L.F., Kem, W.R., Freedman, R. (2004). Alpha-7 nicotinic receptor agonists: potential new candidates for the treatment of schizophrenia. Psychopharmacology, Vol. 174, No. 1, pp. 54-64, ISSN 0033-3158

Martin, S.J., de Hoz, L., Morris, R.G. (2005). Retrograde amnesia: Neither partial nor complete hippocampal lesions in rats result in preferential sparing of remote spatial memory, even after reminding. Neuropsychologia, Vol. 43, pp. 609–624, ISSN 0028-3932

Martin, L.F., Freedman, R. (2007). Schizophrenia and the alpha7 nicotinic acetylcholine receptor. International Review of Neurobiology, Vol. 78, pp. 225-246, ISSN 0074-7742

McNamara, R.K., Skelton, R.W. (1993). The neuropharmacological and neurochemical basis of place learning in the Morris water maze. Brain Research Reviews, Vol. 18, No. 1, pp. :33-49 - ISSN 0165-0173

Mittelstaedt, M.L., Mittelstaedt, H. (1980). Homing by path integration in a mammal. Naturwissenschaften, Vol. 67, pp. 566-567, ISSN 0028-1042

Mittelstaedt, M.L., Glasauer, S. (1991). Idiothetic navigation in gerbils and humans. Zoologische Jahrbücher. Abteilung für allgemeine Zoologie und Physiologie der Tiere, pp. 427-435, ISSN 0044-5185

Moghaddam, M., Bures, J. (1996). Contribution of egocentric spatial memory to place navigation of rats in the Morris water maze. Behavioral Brain Research, Vol. 78, No. 2, pp. 121-129, ISSN 0166-4328

Moghaddam, M., Bures, J. (1997). Rotation of water in the Morris water maze interferes with path integration mechanisms of place navigation. Neurobiology of Learning and Memory, Vol. 68, No. 3, pp. 239-251, ISSN 1074-7427

Morris, R.G.M. (1981). Spatial localization does not require the presence of local cues, Learning and Motivation, Vol. 12, pp. 239-260, ISSN 0023-9690

Morris, R.G.M., Garrud, P., Rawlings, J. and O'Keefe, J. (1982). Place navigation impaired in rats with hippocampal lesions. Nature, Vol. 297, pp. 681-683, ISSN 0028-0836

Morris, R., (1984). Developments of a water-maze procedure for studying spatial learning in the rat, Journal of Neuroscience Methods, Vol. 11, pp. 47-60, ISSN 0165-0270

Morris, R.G., Frey, U. (1997). Hippocampal synaptic plasticity: role in spatial learning or the automatic recording of attended experience? Philosophical Transactions of the Royal Society of London Series B, Vol. 352, No. 1360, pp. 1489-1503, ISSN 0080-4622

Muller, R. (1996). A quarter of a century of place cells. Neuron, Vol. 17, No. 5, pp. 813-822, ISSN 0896-6273

Nekovarova, T., Bures, J. (2006a). Spatial decisions in rats based on the geometry of computer-generated patterns. Neuroscience Letters, Vol. 394, No. 3, pp. 211-215, ISSN 0304-3940

Nekovárová, T., Klement, D. (2006b). Operant behavior of the rat can be controlled by the configuration of objects in an animated scene displayed on a computer screen. Physiological Research, Vol. 55, No. 1, pp. 105-113, ISSN 0862-8408

Nekovarova, T., Nedvidek, J., Bures, J. (2006c). Spatial choices of rats based on abstract visual information: Pattern- or configuration-discrimination? Behavioral Brain Research, Vol. 172, No. 2, pp. 264-271, ISSN 0166-4328

Nekovarova, T., Nedvidek, J., Klement, D., Bures, J. (2009). Spatial decisions and cognitive strategies of monkeys and humans based on abstract spatial stimuli in rotation test. Proceedings of the National Academy of Sciences, USA, Vol. 106, No. 36, pp. 15478-15482, ISSN 0027-8424

O'Carroll, C.M., Martin, S.J., Sandin, J., Frenguelli, B., Morris, R.G. (2006). Dopaminergic modulation of the persistence of one-trial hippocampus-dependent memory. Learning and Memory, Vol. 13, No. 6, pp. 760-769, ISSN 1072-0502

O'Keefe, J. Dostrovsky, J. (1971). The hippocampus as a spatial map. Preliminary evidence from unit activity in the freely moving rat. Brain Research, Vol. 34, pp. 171-175, ISSN 0006-8993

O'Keefe, J., Nadel, L. (1978). The Hippocampus as a Cognitive Map. Clarendon Press, ISBN 0-19-857206-9

Olds, J., Milner, P. (1954). Positive reinforcement produced by by electrical stimulation of septal area. Journal of Comparative & Physiological Psychology, Vol. 47, pp. 419-427, ISSN 0021-9940

Olton, D.S., Samuelson, R.J. (1976). Remembrance of places passed: spatial memory in rats, Journal of Experimental Psychology: Animal Behavior Processes, Vol. 2, pp. 97-116, ISSN 0097-7403

Olton, D.S., Paras, B.C. (1979a). Spatial memory and hippocampal function. Neuropsychologia, Vol. 17, No. 6, pp. 669-682, ISSN 0028-3932

Olton, D.S. (1979b). Mazes, maps, and memory. American Psychologist, Vol. 34, No. 7, pp. 583-596, ISSN 0003-066X

Olton, D.S., Becker, J.T., Handelmann, G.E. (1980). Hippocampal function - working memory or cognitive mapping. Physiological psychology, Vol. 8, No. 2, pp. 239,

Ouagazzal, A., Grottick, A.J., Moreau, J., Higgins, G.A. (2001). Effect of LSD on prepulse inhibition and spontaneous behavior in the rat. A pharmacological analysis and comparison between two rat strains. Neuropsychopharmacology, Vol. 25, No. 4, pp. 565-575, ISSN 0893-133X

Packard, M.G., Hirsh, R., White, N.M. (1989). Differential effects of fornix and caudate nucleus lesions on two radial maze tasks: evidence for multiple memory systems. Journal of Neuroscience, Vol. 9, No. 5, pp. 1465-1472, ISSN 0270-6474

Pálenícek, T., Hlinák, Z., Bubeníková-Valesová, V., Votava, M., Horácek, J. (2007). An analysis of spontaneous behavior following acute MDMA treatment in male and female rats. Neuroendocrinology Letters, Vol. 28, No. 6, pp. 781-788, ISSN 0172-780X

Pálenícek, T., Balíková, M., Bubeníková-Valesová, V., Horácek, J. (2008). Mescaline effects on rat behavior and its time profile in serum and brain tissue after a single subcutaneous dose. Psychopharmacology, Vol. 196, No. 1, pp. 51-62, ISSN 0033-3158

Pastalkova, E., Kelemen, E., Bures, J. (2003). Operant behavior can be triggered by the position of the rat relative to objects rotating on an inaccessible platform. Proceedings of the National Academy of Sciences, USA, Vol. 100, No. 4, pp. 2094-2099, ISSN 0027-8424

Pastalkova, E., Serrano, P., Pinkhasova, D., Wallace, E., Fenton, A.A., Sacktor, T.C. (2006). Storage of spatial information by the maintenance mechanism of LTP. Science. Vol. 313, No. 5790, pp. 1141-1144, ISSN 0036-8075

Powell, S.B., Zhou, X., Geyer, M.A. (2009). Prepulse inhibition and genetic mouse models of schizophrenia. Behavioral Brain Research, Vol. 204, No. 2, pp. 282-294, ISSN 0166-4328

Rambousek, L., Bubenikova-Valesova, V., Kacer, P., Syslova, K., Kenney, J., Holubova, K., Najmanova, V., Zach, P., Svoboda, J., Stuchlik, A., Chodounska, H., Kapras, V., Adamusova, E., Borovska, J., Vyklicky, L., Vales, K. (2011). Cellular and behavioural effects of a new steroidal inhibitor of the N-methyl-d-aspartate receptor 3α5β-pregnanolone glutamate. Neuropharmacology, Vol. 61, No. 1-2, pp. 61-6, ISSN 0028-3908

Rezacova, L., Svoboda, J., Stuchlik, A., Vales, K. (2011). Differential effects of stable elevated levels of corticotropin-releasing hormone and systemic corticosterone on various types of rat learning. Neuroendocrinology Letters, Vol. 32, No. 1, pp. 64-76, ISSN 0172-780X

Rich, B.A., Vinton, D., Grillon, C., Bhangoo, R.K., Leibenluft, E. (2005). An investigation of prepulse inhibition in pediatric bipolar disorder. Bipolar Disorders, Vol. 7, No. 2, pp. 198-203, ISSN 1398-5647

Sams-Dodd, F., Lipska, B.K., Weinberger, D.R. (1997). Neonatal lesions of the rat ventral hippocampus result in hyperlocomotion and deficits in social behaviour in adulthood. Psychopharmacology, Vol. 132, No. 3, pp. 303-310, ISSN 0033-3158

Saucier, D., Hargreaves, E.L., Boon, F., Vanderwolf, C.H., Cain, D.P. (1996). Detailed behavioral analysis of water maze acquisition under systemic NMDA or muscarinic antagonism: nonspatial pretraining eliminates spatial learning deficits. Behavioral Neuroscience, Vol. 110, No. 1, pp. 103-116, ISSN 0735-7044

Sharma, S., Rakoczy, S., Brown-Borg, H. (2010). Assessment of spatial memory in mice. Life Science, Vol. 87, No. 17-18, pp. 521-536, ISSN 0024-3205

Skarsfeldt, T. (1996). Differential effect of antipsychotics on place navigation of rats in the Morris water maze. A comparative study between novel and reference antipsychotics. Psychopharmacology, Vol. 124, No. 1-2, pp. 126-133, ISSN 0033-3158

Solstad, T., Boccara, C.N., Kropff, E., Moser, M.B., Moser, E.I. (2008). Representation of geometric borders in the entorhinal cortex. Science, Vol. 322, No. 5909, pp. 1865-1868, ISSN 0036-8075

Spooner, R.I., Thomson, A., Hall, J., Morris, R.G., Salter, S.H. (1994). The Atlantis platform: a new design and further developments of Buresova's on-demand platform for the water maze. Learning and Memory, Vol. 1, No. 3, pp. 203-211, ISSN 1072-0502

Steele, R.J., Morris, R.G. (1999). Delay-dependent impairment of a matching-to-place task with chronic and intrahippocampal infusion of the NMDA-antagonist D-AP5. Hippocampus, Vol. 9, No. 2, pp. 118-136, ISSN 1050-9631

Stuchlik, A., Fenton, A.A., Bures, J. (2001). Substratal idiothetic navigation of rats is impaired by removal or devaluation of extramaze and intramaze cues. Proceedings of the National Academy of Sciences, USA, Vol. 98, No. 6, pp. 3537-3542, ISSN 0027-8424

Stuchlik, A., Bures, J. (2002). Relative contribution of allothetic and idiothetic navigation to place avoidance on stable and rotating arenas in darkness. Behavioral Brain Research, Vol. 128, No. 2, pp. 179-188, ISSN 0166-4328

Stuchlik, A., Rezacova, L., Vales, K., Bubenikova, V., Kubik, S. (2004). Application of a novel Active Allothetic Place Avoidance task (AAPA) in testing a pharmacological model of psychosis in rats: comparison with the Morris Water Maze. Neuroscience Letters, Vol. 366, No. 2, pp. 162-166, ISSN 0304-3940

Stuchlík, A., Vales, K. (2005). Systemic administration of MK-801, a non-competitive NMDA-receptor antagonist, elicits a behavioural deficit of rats in the Active Allothetic Place Avoidance (AAPA) task irrespectively of their intact spatial pretraining. Behavioral Brain Research, Vol. 159, No. 1, pp. 163-171, ISSN 0166-4328

Stuchlik, A., Rehakova, L., Telensky, P., Vales, K. (2007a). Morris water maze learning in Long-Evans rats is differentially affected by blockade of D1-like and D2-like dopamine receptors. Neuroscience Letters, Vol. 422, No. 3, pp. 169-174, ISSN 0304-3940

Stuchlik, A., Rehakova, L., Rambousek, L., Svoboda, J., Vales, K. (2007b). Manipulation of D2 receptors with quinpirole and sulpiride affects locomotor activity before spatial behavior of rats in an active place avoidance task. Neuroscience Research, Vol. 58, No. 2, pp. 133-139, ISSN 0168-0102

Stuchlík, A., Petrásek, T., Vales, K. (2009). Effect of alpha(1)-adrenergic antagonist prazosin on behavioral alterations induced by MK-801 in a spatial memory task in Long-Evans rats. Physiological Research, Vol. 58, No. 5, pp. 733-740, ISSN 0862-8408

Stuchlik, A., Petrasek, T., Prokopova, I., Bahnik, S., Berger, S., Schonig K., Vales, K., Bartsch, D. (2011). Genetic neurodevelopmental models in biological psychiatry: A study of hippocampusdependent learning in rats with neuronal nogo– a knockdown - Free

Communication FC-17-002, 10th World Congress of Biological Psychiatry, Prague, http://www.wfsbp-congress.org

Svoboda, J., Telensky, P., Blahna, K., Zach, P., Bures, J., Stuchlik, A. (2008). Lesion of posterior parietal cortex in rats does not disrupt place avoidance based on either distal or proximal orienting cues. Neuroscience Letters, Vol. 445, No. 1, pp. 73-77, ISSN 0304-3940

Swerdlow, N.R., Braff, D.L., Geyer, M.A., Koob, G.F. (1986). Central dopamine hyperactivity in rats mimics abnormal acoustic startle response in schizophrenics. Biological Psychiatry, Vol. 21, No. 1, pp. 23-33, ISSN 0006-3223

Swerdlow, N.R., Weber, M., Qu, Y., Light, G.A., Braff, D.L. (2008). Realistic expectations of prepulse inhibition in translational models for schizophrenia research. Psychopharmacology, Vol. 199, No. 3, pp. 331-388, ISSN 0033-3158

Szechtman, H., Eckert, M.J., Tse, W.S., Boersma, J.T., Bonura, C.A., McClelland, J.Z., Culver, K.E., Eilam, D. (2001). Compulsive checking behavior of quinpirole-sensitized rats as an animal model of Obsessive-Compulsive Disorder(OCD): form and control. BMC Neuroscience, Vol. 2, pp. 4, ISSN 1471-2202

Taube, J.S., Muller, R.U., Ranck, J.B. (1990a) Head direction cells recorded from the postsubiculum in freely moving rats I. Description and quantitative analysis, Journal of Neuroscience, Vol. 10, pp. 420-435, ISSN 0270-6474

Taube, J.S., Muller, R.U., Ranck, J.B. (1990b) Head direction cells recorded from the postsubiculum in freely moving rats II. The effects of environmental manipulations, Journal of Neuroscience, Vol. 10, pp. 436-447, ISSN 0270-6474

Telensky, P., Svoboda, J., Blahna, K., Bureš, J., Kubik, S., Stuchlik, A. (2011). Functional inactivation of the rat hippocampus disrupts avoidance of a moving object. Proceedings of the National Academy of Sciences, USA, Vol. 108, No. 13, pp. 5414-5418, ISSN 0027-8424

Telensky, P., Svoboda, J., Pastalkova, E., Blahna, K., Bures, J., Stuchlik, A. (2009). Enemy avoidance task: a novel behavioral paradigm for assessing spatial avoidance of a moving subject. Journal of Neuroscience Methods, Vol. 180, No. 1, pp. 29-33, ISSN 0165-0270

Thomsen, M., Wess, J., Fulton, B.S., Fink-Jensen, A., Caine, S.B. (2010). Modulation of prepulse inhibition through both M(1) and M (4) muscarinic receptors in mice. Psychopharmacology, Vol. 208, No. 3, pp. 401-416, ISSN 0033-3158

Tordjman, S., Drapier, D., Bonnot, O., Graignic, R., Fortes, S., Cohen, D., Millet, B., Laurent, C., Roubertoux, P.L. (2007). Animal models relevant to schizophrenia and autism: validity and limitations. Behavior Genetics, Vol. 37, No. 1, pp. 61-78, ISSN: 0001-8244

Ueki, A., Goto, K., Sato, N., Iso, H., Morita, Y. (2006). Prepulse inhibition of acoustic startle response in mild cognitive impairment and mild dementia of Alzheimer type. Psychiatry and Clinical Neurosciences, Vol. 60, No. 1, pp. 55-62, online ISSN 1440-1819

Vales, K., Stuchlik, A. (2005). Central muscarinic blockade interferes with retrieval and reacquisition of active allothetic place avoidance despite spatial pretraining. Behavioral Brain Research, Vol. 161, No. 2, pp. 238-244, ISSN 0166-4328

Vales, K., Bubenikova-Valesova, V., Klement, D., Stuchlik, A. (2006). Analysis of sensitivity to MK-801 treatment in a novel active allothetic place avoidance task and in the working memory version of the Morris water maze reveals differences between Long-Evans and Wistar rats. Neuroscience Research, Vol. 55, No. 4, pp. 383-388, ISSN 0168-0102

Vales, K., Svoboda, J., Benkovicova, K., Bubenikova-Valesova, V., Stuchlik, A. (2010). The difference in effect of mGlu2/3 and mGlu5 receptor agonists on cognitive impairment induced by MK-801. European Journal of Pharmacology, Vol. 639, No. 1-3, pp. 91-98, ISSN 0014-2999

van den Buuse, M. (2010). Modeling the positive symptoms of schizophrenia in genetically modified mice: pharmacology and methodology aspects. Schizophrenia Bulletin, Vol. 36, No. 2, pp. 246-270, ISSN 0586-7614

van der Staay, F.J., Rutten, K., Erb, C., Blokland, A. (2011). Effects of the cognition impairer MK-801 on learning and memory in mice and rats. Behavioral Brain Research, Vol. 220, No. 1, pp. 215-229, ISSN 0166-4328

Van Snellenberg, J.X. (2009). Working memory and long-term memory deficits in schizophrenia: is there a common substrate? Psychiatry Research, Vol. 174, No. 2, pp. 89-96, ISSN 0165-1781

Wesierska, M., Adamska, I., Malinowska, M. (2009). Retrosplenial cortex lesion affected segregation of spatial information in place avoidance task in the rat. Neurobiology of Learning and Memory, Vol. 91, No. 1, pp. 41-49, ISSN 1074-7427

Wesierska, M., Dockery, C., Fenton, A.A. (2005). Beyond memory, navigation, and inhibition: behavioral evidence for hippocampus-dependent cognitive coordination in the rat. Journal of Neuroscience, Vol. 25, No. 9, pp. 2413-2419, ISSN 0270-6474

Woody, E.Z., Szechtman, H. (2011). Adaptation to potential threat: the evolution, neurobiology, and psychopathology of the security motivation system. Neuroscience and Biobehavioral Reviews, Vol. 35, No. 4, pp. 1019-1033, ISSN 0149-7634

Zeldin, R.K., Olton, D.S. (1986). Rats acquire spatial learning sets. Journal of Experimental Psychology: Animal Behavior Processes, Vol. 12, No. 4, pp. 412-419. ISSN 0097-7403

Zhuravin, I.A., Bures, J. (1991). Extent of the tetrodotoxin induced blockade examined by pupillary paralysis elicited by intracerebral injection of the drug. Experimental Brain Research, Vol. 83, No. 3, pp. 687-690, ISSN 0014-4819